THE VERTUE METHOD

SHONA VERTUE

THE VERTUE METHOD

A stronger, fitter, healthier you – in 28 days

Photography by Helen Cathcart and Leo Cackett

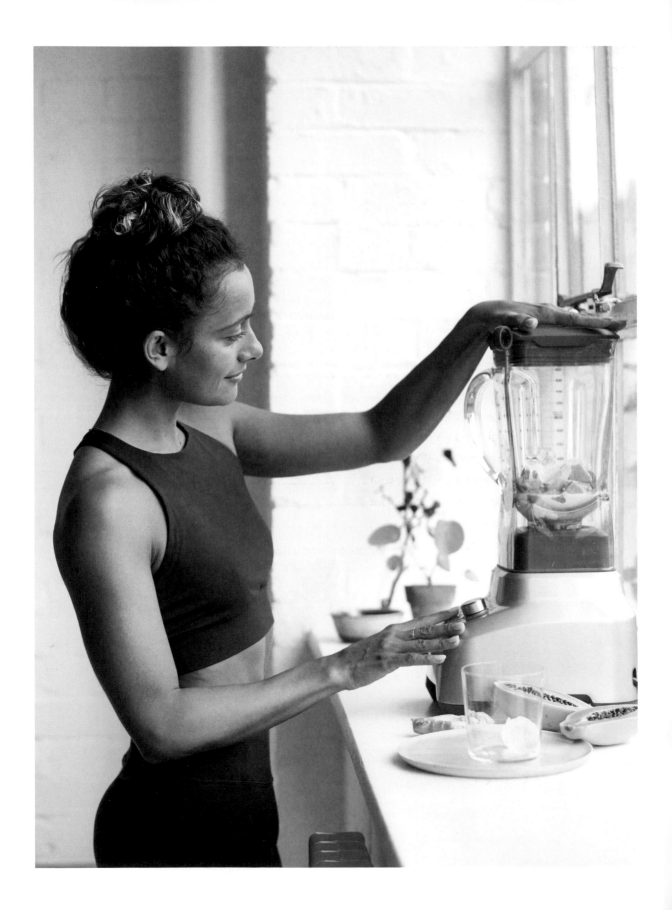

CONTENTS

INTRODUCTION

I'm no psychic, but I'm guessing that you have picked up this book in an effort to become healthier, stronger, fitter, leaner or more toned. Great. You've chosen the right book, or perhaps this book chose you. I often feel that books find their way into our lives just at the right time, don't you?

My intention behind writing this book was to start a revolution. I want you to get healthier, stronger, fitter and more toned but, more importantly, I want to kick-start a massive revolution in the way that you approach your health and fitness practices so that you will keep them going forever.

Are you someone who has tried every fitness class out there... once... but nothing has ever really stuck? Are you someone who gets to the gym and doesn't know what to do once you're there? Or perhaps you could run a 10K but can barely touch your toes? Are you diligent about making it to your Monday night yoga class but couldn't do a full chin-up?

If you answered yes to any of the above, then this book is for you.

When it comes to health, many of us can fall into the trap of practising the things that we're already pretty good at, while avoiding the things our bodies need. The Vertue Method combines the philosophies of various training modalities which help to bring about a sustainable and healthy balance within your body and life.

Getting fit, for most of us, is usually motivated by the aesthetic benefits it can bring. We all want to feel attractive. However, I believe – actually I know – that the secret to achieving long-lasting, sustainable visual results is falling in love with all of the other benefits that fitness and health can bring too. Benefits such as being able to run up an escalator without gasping for air, doing push-ups and pull-ups with ease, being stronger, feeling badass, primal, capable, wild and, above all, FREE. Yes – a good training and nutritional practice can make you feel that good.

This book is going to remind you of all the reasons to take care of your body, while getting you stronger, more flexible and more at peace in mind and body. Of course it will help you to achieve that leaner, fitter, chiselled, toned, sculpted body you have been wanting, but not at the cost of your health or happiness.

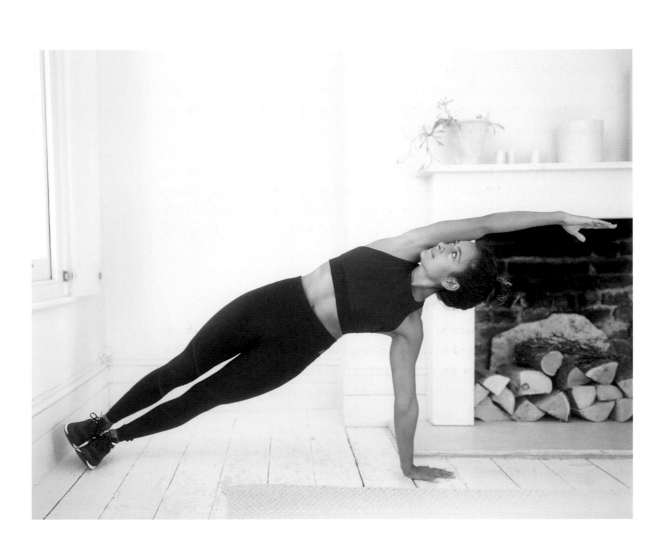

MY VERTUEOUS STORY

When my parents enrolled me in gymnastics at the age of four, I would never have imagined that a few years later I would be training a total of 20 hours a week, before and after school and at weekends. Innocently jumping around on a trampoline, excited and wide-eyed, with my heart pounding through my teeny toddler chest, I had no idea that by nine years old I would be taking trips to the Australian Institute of Sport in Canberra to audition as a potential recruit for the Olympic team.

For years I lived and breathed the sport. However, with secondary school fast approaching my mother and father sat me down one day and asked me if I wanted to do gymnastics full-time or stay in school, and although I was only 12 years old, I knew in my heart that I did not want a career in gymnastics. Sadly, it isn't a sport you can dabble in, so I chose school and quit gymnastics.

I took the movement skills I had acquired from gymnastics into dance and successfully auditioned as a dancer for the Newtown High School of the Performing Arts and there moved into all forms of performing arts – dance, drama and music.

Although movement was a part of my daily life, it was nowhere near as rigorous as my gymnastics conditioning regime. My father became concerned that the reduction in activity meant that I was going to lose the athletic strength and build that I had developed while training as an elite gymnast, and so doing what he thought was best, he enrolled me into the local gym and we would train side by side for an hour every morning before school.

Something interesting shifted during this period of my life: my motivation for training. As a gymnast I eagerly awoke to my alarm because it meant getting closer to that backflip or back somersault or even triple back somersault in the gym. It was fun, it was challenging and it had a wonderful, life-enriching purpose. But when I began training in the gym, mindlessly pushing and pulling machines, I lost that sense of purpose. I was suddenly training only to maintain some kind of ideal aesthetic physique, rather than training to develop or condition a skill. I began using the physiques of other beautiful, slim women in magazines and on TV to motivate me to train, rather than looking to skilful athletes and their abilities. It was a subtle but important shift in my psyche and one that would teach me some important lessons on the difference between fitness and health. I believe that at some point in our young adulthood a lot of us will go through a sad transition, from running around the park because it's fun, to running around the park because if we don't move enough we will get fat. I truly believe that with this loss of joy lies one of the biggest barriers to health, wellness and even weight loss.

When I finished secondary school I had no idea what I wanted to do – my passion was deeply rooted in the performing arts, but I also wanted to earn money (unfortunately these two things don't always come hand in hand for everyone!). Knowing that with money comes freedom, I applied for a secretarial role and began an intense but short-lived stint as an executive assistant.

Sitting behind a desk for eight hours a day just wasn't for me, and it generally made me feel pretty depressed. I didn't appreciate just how sad I was – or how I was using food, especially sugar, as a means to distract myself from the discomfort and self-perpetuating vexation with my situation. My skin was bad, I was tired all the time and I found myself in hospital several times with gastroenteritis. This sadness also caused me to neglect exercise. The lack of movement itself would have played a huge part in the development of the sadness. One reinforces the other – a vicious and all too common cycle.

In many eastern philosophies they say that suffering is our greatest teacher, and in my case it was this time of illness in both body and mind that brought me to one of the greatest pleasures in my life: yoga. I went to a yoga class in Sydney and it was love at first sun salutation. I recognised immediately the healing powers of the practice and began to research it further. I felt a stirring of the feelings I used to have while doing gymnastics, and quickly became hooked.

I soon wanted to share what I was learning through yoga with those around me. I wanted to start teaching what I was preaching. I took a leap of faith, quit my much-disliked job and started my life as a more or less destitute yoga teacher. The money (or lack thereof) didn't matter. I was so happy to have found what felt like my calling.

During this time I was still going to the gym – all those mornings training with my dad had instilled a habit and I still hopped on the treadmill regularly and used the machines, although I would mostly try to distract myself by watching TV shows. While working as a yoga teacher in some prominent gyms in Sydney, I had the

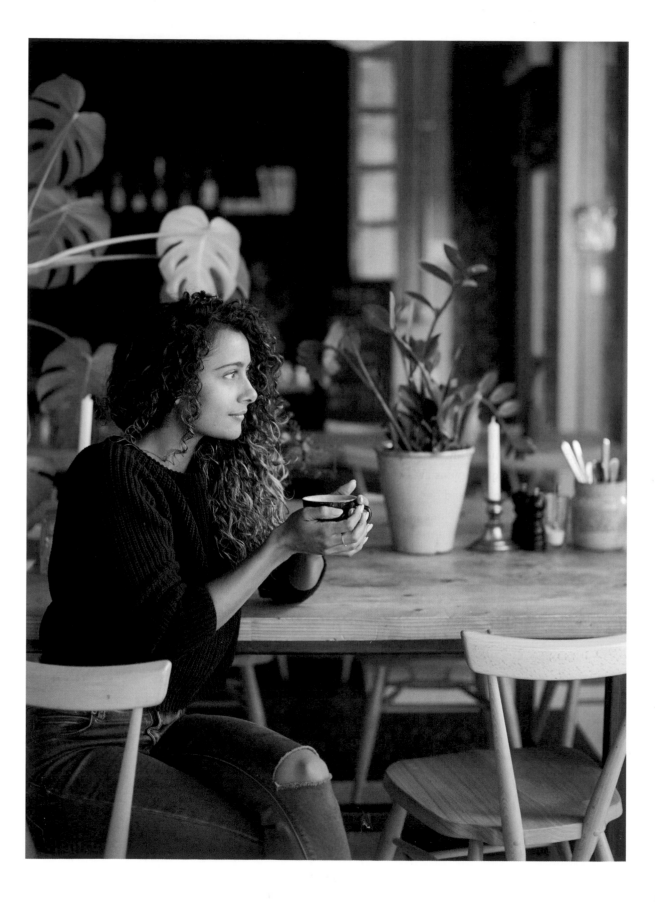

privilege of meeting some incredible trainers and teachers and, as I became immersed in the fitness industry, my workouts began to shift in style. I learned about the benefits of weight lifting for women, and gradually spent less time on the machines and more time with the dumb-bells.

I noted the profound effect weight lifting was having on both my body shape and my yoga practice. I could hold handstands for longer and take on arm balances I never ever thought possible. Most of all, I felt extremely powerful, with a new-found feeling of strength growing within my body. In addition to this my arms took on the shape I had been longing for, my abs formed elegantly and my butt grew (higher not wider).

Weight lifting became my new addiction. It filled the physical strength gaps that I felt yoga was missing. I felt sexier and had fewer aches and injuries, and it was really all down to the strength I was developing within the weights room.

I wanted to share this new fitness passion with my clients; I wanted to show people the benefits of combining both strength and flexibility training. I completed my personal training certificate and was lucky enough to become a personal trainer at one of the most prestigious gyms in Sydney. I found myself surrounded by the best personal trainers in the city and became a sponge for all their incredible experience and knowledge. It was honestly one of the biggest and most important learning curves of my life.

Here's where my story takes a slightly strange, brief turn. I am quite a small person and all that time around people in the fitness industry left me feeling somewhat intimidated by the big and strong personal trainers (both male and female). They lifted more, grew more and knew more than me, and I was insecure because of it. I wanted to prove my self-worth in that gym environment and so started bodybuilding and entering competitions.

It was a very intense journey and I will never do it again! Yet I was taught some valuable lessons and won the competitions that I took part in. I learned about diet, fat loss and muscle gain – but I would say that, more importantly, I came to understand the damaging effects of placing your entire sense of self-worth on how you appear aesthetically. Bodybuilding and fitness competing have you focusing on every inch, or even millimetre, of fat on your body, and the less fat you have, the more likely you are to win. There are other components to it of course, but all the criteria are heavily based around physical appearance – it's extremely pernicious and creeps up on you when you least expect it.

When I quit bodybuilding, I felt a little lost with my training, my nutrition and my entire life direction. I knew I wasn't going to be a professional athlete and I wanted to experience a challenge that would be greater than just shifting body fat or being flexible. I wanted to explore and become more cultured, and I wanted to get out of my lovely – but somewhat vacuous – existence in Bondi; a place with such an infectious atmosphere and hypnotic energy that it can be very hard to leave. But I knew that if I wanted to grow as a person, I would have to venture to other worlds.

I chose London.

It might seem obvious, but I was kind of surprised when I arrived by how much less people exercised in London than in Sydney. However, it also made sense that with a nine-month cold season, a two-week summer and a couple of months in between spent in rainy limbo, the whole idea of bikini aesthetics didn't really apply in the same way. People spend most of their lives under multiple layers of clothes and a big coat. I get it! A rainy day in Sydney would always result in a busy gym; a rainy day in London results in a busy pub.

I had to adapt my approach and search for different ways to give purpose to my clients' workouts. I started to use words emphasising their strength- and skill-based goals rather than simply 'let's burn some calories'! I demanded they focus their attention on increasing numbers on the dumb-bells, rather than reducing digits on the scales. The more they lifted in the gym, provided they were adequately nourished, the less body fat they carried.

Interestingly, the less they focused on those aesthetic goals the easier they seemed to find it to eat healthy food. They said they didn't feel like they were restricting themselves to get thin; instead they WANTED to make healthy choices so that they would train harder and lift more in the gym. Suddenly dieting was about nourishing, not punishing.

Moving to the UK has had an incredibly profound effect on my training ethos, and has played a big role in my approach to fitness and health. Although many associate a trip to London as a pub-crawling party to the Heathrow Injection*, the Vertue Method would not have been created without being exposed to life here. Despite my hourly complaints about the weather, I am so deeply grateful for all that the UK has taught me so far, and I am even more grateful to be able to share this Method with you, in an effort to help you find the balance you require to feel truly healthy and wildly free.

*For those that aren't aware, the Heathrow Injection is essentially a metaphor for the 'inevitable' weight that foreigners gain after moving to London – usually from a winter-warming diet of lager, Yorkshire puddings, pies and Hobnobs.

THE VERTUE METHOD

WHAT IS THE VERTUE METHOD?

The Vertue Method is an approach to wellness that came about as the culmination of my experience as an elite gymnast, dancer, personal trainer and yoga teacher. It is a practice that places equal importance on developing strength and flexibility, and nourishing the body and mind with nutritious food and consistent meditation practices.

To me, a healthy body needs to be both strong and flexible. However, we live in a fairly time-poor society – or at least it seems that way – and I have found that the people I have come across while working as a trainer in London tend to neglect either their strength training or their stretching (and sometimes both!).

The Vertue Method approach was created with these time-poor people in mind. I honestly thought that I knew what 'busy' meant when I was working in Sydney, and then I moved to London... and learned the true meaning of the word. My client base in London has ranged from lawyers to lab assistants, from stay-at-home dads to single working mothers – and while their daily lives differ immensely, one similarity remains: they are all busy AF. The only way I could ensure they all worked on strength, flexibility and meditation was to make sure that we did it all in the session. The body doesn't care if you're busy; it still requires love and care. Give it the right kind of care and it will help you continue to be busy doing the things you want to do, chasing the dreams that you want to achieve.

At the risk of stating the obvious, strong muscles and supportive joints are pretty damn important and, likewise, being able to move those strong joints and muscles freely is also vital. To support the achievement of this strong yet agile body we need to nourish it properly. It is for this reason that the Vertue Method is an approach to health and wellness that holds equilibrium in the utmost importance.

To achieve this harmony, the Vertue Method is divided into three pillars:

LIFT (things that are heavier than a handbag to grow muscle and build strength)

LENGTHEN (your spine and free your joints using daily yoga and mobility practices)

NOURISH (both your body and mind with wholesome food and meditation)

These three things have shaped my body and my life, as well as the bodies and lives of my clients. By broadening your knowledge of wellness through these pillars, I know that you will also experience a transformation that far surpasses just looking 'hotter' at the beach.

My 28-day reset plan is the perfect way for you to begin to integrate the Vertue Method into your own life. Over the course of the 28 days you're going to be completing six workouts a week. Four of those workouts will be weighted; the other two will be cardio-focused. In addition to the intense physical activity, each night you will also be following one of two sequences that will help you increase your mobility and flexibility while also aiding your body to relax and unwind before bed. One of these sequences uses a mobility ball to release muscle tension; the other is a yoga-based sequence that will help you to increase your flexibility.

To support all this exercise, you are going to nourish your body and mind. I have provided a 28-day food plan (with accompanying recipes) for you to follow, along with three different meditation options that you will practise every morning to help you nurture your mind.

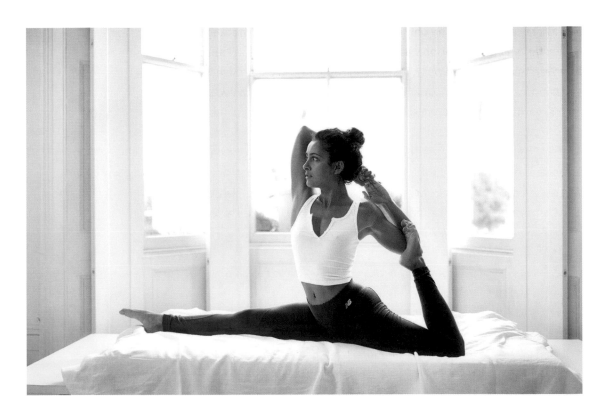

Before you embark on all that I want you to get through the 'philosophy' and 'knowledge' section of the book first. I understand that there is quite a large load of information to digest, but I believe that understating the 'why' can help to motivate you far more than just being told what to do. So do your best to absorb, understand and apply the information from the three pillars before embarking on the reset plan.

THE PROMISE

Stronger, leaner, fitter and more energised are just a few of the words that will describe you upon finishing the 28-day reset plan. However, the best and most important part of all of it is how good you will feel!

At the moment there is a growing trend, particularly in cities, towards boot-camps and militant-style high intensity interval training (HIIT) sessions. HIIT is a form of cardiovascular training that uses highly demanding movements to get your heart rate very high, with minimal rest periods. It can be effective for fat burning, but is very taxing on the nervous system. For most of these sessions the focus is placed on intensity and challenge. However, as you'll discover as you go through this book, fatigue and sweat are not necessarily correlational to results.

While there is nothing wrong with the occasional HIIT workout, using these styles as your main or only form of training can be more damaging than you think. If the most active part of your day is getting in and out of a hammock, or taking an afternoon stroll by the sea, then yes, potentially HIIT every morning could be suitable. However, for those of us living in bustling cities that move faster than the speed of a British summer, adding yet another highly stressful form of exercise on top of an already stressful life is not favourable to developing long-term results, or true health. In fact, it can hinder results. Excess cortisol has been shown to inhibit fat loss and even cause the storage of fat around the tummy. In the same way that you can't out-train a bad diet, you can't out-train a stressful lifestyle.

The Vertue Method workouts always begin and end with a meditational focus on the breath and body, to leave you feeling calm but uplifted (which is why the Vertue Method uplifts your soul and your butt). And although challenging, the workouts place great emphasis on controlled and precise movement, ensuring that you will achieve results safely and effectively.

When it comes to food, I know that many people often believe that they have to suffer in order to see results, but what if I told you that you could get the body you've always wanted without having to live off steamed fish and broccoli, do intense cardio on an empty stomach, take 120 different supplements or drink a green juice that tastes like your back garden?

The Vertue Method acknowledges that we are lovers of pleasure, and so why should our approach to fitness and food be any different? The Vertue Method plan promises to provide you with the tools and techniques to emancipate a balanced and therefore healthier body and mind in a way that helps you to *enjoy the process*. It is designed to help you cultivate the balance required both physically and mentally so that you can continue to do the things you love, while also sculpting the body of your dreams.

The truth is that there are many ways to achieve a toned, lean and athletic body, but the most successful, sustainable and effective process is the one you enjoy. We all want results, but we are hindered usually by two things: time and enjoyment factor. The Vertue Method workouts are between 25 and 45 minutes. I personally don't have time for 90-minute workouts and I'm assuming you don't either, so my workouts have been designed to get you maximal results in minimal time. I don't believe you need to work more than 45 minutes, and research suggests that working over that can induce stress. By the same token, 25 minutes is the minimum, because I don't believe in any training fad that promises results by doing only 15 minutes of exercise a day.

The Vertue Method acknowledges that we are lovers of pleasure, and so why should our approach to fitness and food be any different?

Joy is a huge but often underrated aspect of a fitness regime, and that is where the philosophy of the Vertue Method plays a big part. Aside from developing a leaner and more sculpted body, there are very specific skill-based exercises that will keep your mind invested in the practice. Having toned arms is great, but having toned arms that can hold you in a handstand or perform a full push-up boosts training motivation to the next level, because it's both functional and fun.

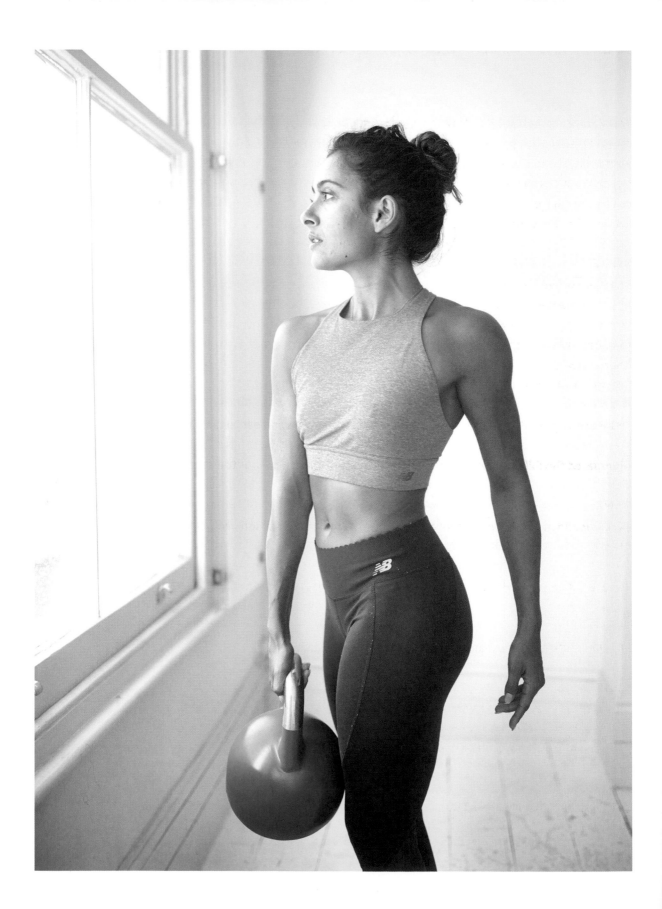

The Vertue Method is a new way to approach your health regime, and because of this it won't just change your mind and body, it will change your life. It will strengthen your ability to do those things that make you excited for life, because I believe that health practices should enhance your life, not take away from it. The Vertue Method has been created with this as a core principle. Some of the changes that you can expect to see in your body and mind upon completion of the 28-day reset plan are:

BODY

- **Leaner:** in four weeks of the Vertue Method my clients have reduced their body fat by significant amounts.

- **Increased muscle definition and tone:** this is a common benefit of getting leaner, but also of developing muscle. Simply getting skinny alone will not help you develop shape – weights and correct nutrition build shape.

- **Stronger:** again, this is what happens when you lift weights and eat to nourish.

- **Increased flexibility:** you'll be able to reach for more than just your toes.

MIND

- **Calmer** and much cooler: I'm referring to your temper; meditation can help to reduce the anxiety that leads to angry outbursts.

- **Improved concentration:** consistent meditation practice has been shown to improve concentration.

- **Better attitude:** particularly towards your eating; no more yo-yo shame and binging.

- **Reduced stress.** We can't change the stressful things that happen in our lives, and it's taken me years of trying to control things to realise that the only thing I have control over is how I choose to react to events. The Vertue Method will help you to react in a way that will make it easier for your brain and body to cope

This programme will teach you how to love your body, your butt, exercise, healthy food and even meditation, so that you are successful in attaining the results you desire, for life.

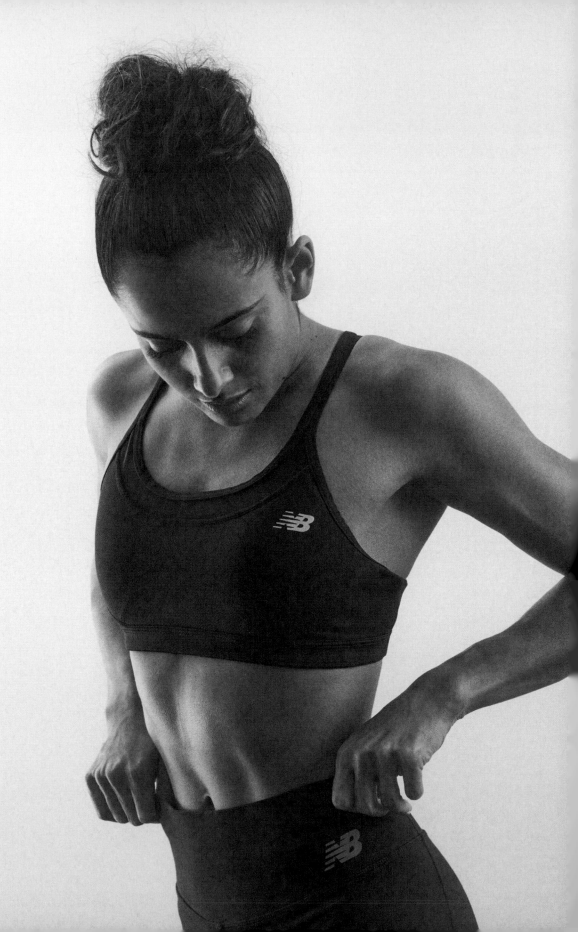

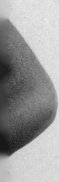

LIFT

LIFT

WHY LIFT?

Introducing weights into my fitness regime changed my shape, my yoga practice, my body composition, my confidence and my headspace – I guess it changed my life.

While there are certainly plenty of incredible bodies out there that train without weights, including gymnasts and dancers who usually only train using their body weight, I believe that lifting weights is a really efficient way to get both the body and the body confidence you want.

I want you to fall in LOVE with training and the empowerment it can liberate from within you. Strengthening your body gives you that Bee Gees' Stayin' Alive kind of spring in your step (if you're too young for a Bee Gees reference, think Beyoncé-level swag). Being strong physically is a confidence booster like nothing else.

Firstly, before I bust this myth, I actually want to say that I do understand what you mean when you say 'bulky'. A lot of women don't like the look of mountainous trapezius muscles sitting atop their shoulders. In addition to this, lots of women don't want big quadzilla thighs or hulking pecs, because they feel as though those sorts of muscles are associated with a more masculine physique and, ultimately, 'bulkiness'.

However, I want to assert to you that you can grow the 'right' type of muscle to develop your 'right' kind of shape. In the Vertue Method I focus on activating your glutes (rather than relying on the quads), working your triceps (rather than your pecs) and maintaining flexibility and awareness of posture to ensure that you develop the shape that you desire.

THINK HEAVY, GET LEAN

A little side note for the women here: nothing peeves me off more than exercise methods that encourage women to lift no heavier than 1.5kg. Not only is it completely impractical – most things that women need to lift on a daily basis weigh more than 1.5kg – but it's also anti-feminist and kind of demeaning! Put down the pink 1lb (500g) dumb-bell and get ready to reap the benefits of picking up a 10kg, cast iron kettlebell. No, you will not become bulky, you will become femininely badass.

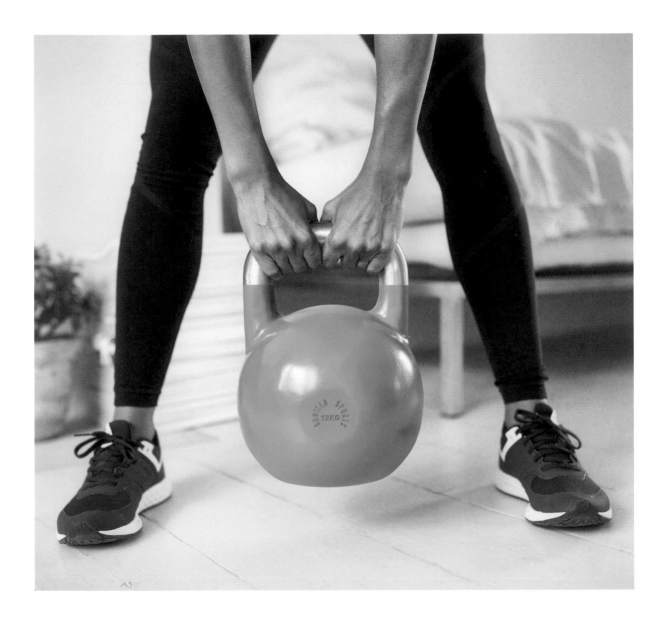

One of the main goals that I have with this book is to debunk the misconceptions there are around growing muscle, and ghostbust the hell out of the fear women have around lifting heavier things. Bottom line: growing muscle is good. Let's just be clever about the ones we choose to grow. Form is key.

MY TOP TEN REASONS TO LIFT MORE WEIGHT

1. Reduced fat – Resistance training isn't just about building muscle. It can also aid in fat loss. There are many studies out there that highlight the benefits that resistance training can have on improving metabolic function and improving fat loss rate[1]. Cardio is still an effective form of fat loss. However, it doesn't do a great job of preserving muscle. By training weights, you also avoid the potential of being just skinny without supporting musculature. Saggy bums are sad bums.

2. Reduced pain – Yes please! I mean, what's not to love about that? Weight lifting has been shown to create profound improvements to the musculoskeletal system, including reduced lower back pain, and prevention of osteoporosis and sarcopenia[2] (muscle loss as a result of ageing).

3. Strong curves and a sexy shape – A good weight-training programme (coupled with the right nutrition) will increase muscle mass, which not only helps us to become stronger (and therefore feel more powerful), but also helps to develop a more defined and athletic shape. Weights create the shape – the right diet will reveal it.

4. To be the boss of glucose – Type 2 diabetes is a metabolic condition in which the pancreas does not produce enough insulin, or the body doesn't react to the insulin produced, leading to the unhealthy rise of blood sugar levels. There have been numerous studies to highlight the benefits of progressive resistance training in those with Type 2 diabetes, including the reduction of blood sugar levels and an increase in muscle glycogen stores – the more that muscle stores glycogen, the less glucose there will be floating around in the blood potentially creating all kinds of havoc[3].

5. Fitter faster – More efficient results. In my experience both as a trainer and trainee, weight training just speeds up the process. As a gymnast I trained using explosive movements and with only my body weight for resistance and I was super strong. However, I trained for 20 hours a week. That's almost a full-time job! Weight lifting has helped me to develop a strong body in a quarter of the time.

6. Feel GOOD! – You don't have to just take my word for it, there are studies (in both the young and elderly) that show the potential psychological benefits of resistance training too, including reduced anxiety, somatisation, depression and hostility[4].

7. Improved flexibility and yoga practices – Yep! This one was probably unexpected, but it's one of my favourite reasons to lift weights. The movements within the Vertue Method plan encourage a full range of movement throughout the joints, while still under load. This actually helps to build flexibility and mobility, without losing strength and stability.

8. Tone – I'm here to break it to you that when you use the word 'toning' you are referring to dropping body fat and increasing muscle mass (slightly). Correct weight training can do both.

9. Healthy goals – We all want to achieve goals and see the results of those goals; it's one of the most motivating factors of exercising. What I love about weight training is that it can help to shift the focus of your goals towards achieving a skill, rather than just simply 'looking better'.

We have to accept the reality that, as humans, the way we look is always going to fluctuate and change. Menstrual cycles, work, break-ups, stress, etc. all affect our weight and our appearance. The best thing about focusing your training goals towards a skill is that it's rarely affected by these events. Gaining a few extra pounds because you've been a little stressed at work is not going to affect your motivation to nail that push-up or pull-up. If you focus on lifting a little heavier each week, you will always feel motivated to train because it's not about how you look, but instead how badass you feel. A weighted dead lift will help you to feel pretty superhero-esque.

10. A better butt – Look, of course there are plenty of ways to develop wonderful glutes, and genetics will often play a part, but I'm going to let you in on a secret. I had the FLATTEST BUTT ever! Nothing, and I mean NOTHING, improved my booty the way that weight training did. The Vertue Method puts a lot of emphasis on developing and sculpting strong and sexy gluteals – more on that later.

BEFORE YOU LIFT

Allrighty, before we even get started on the lifts, I want to give you some information that I believe is important to understand before you even adjust your grip on the pull-up bar. I know there is a lot of information already out there and you are probably raring to get started, but all the writing below is ESSENTIAL to developing your desired body. I don't just want you to take my word for it and I don't just want you to do what I tell you. I want you to understand it so you can be the master of your own booty (and destiny).

MUSCLES

We want them, we use them, we train them and Arnie had a lot of them, but seriously, what actually IS a muscle?

Muscles are divided into three categories within the body: smooth, cardiac and skeletal. Skeletal muscle is what we're going to be most concerned with and is the one that is most responsible for making you look good naked.

Skeletal muscles are connected to the skeleton (no way, really?), and they are part of the mechanical system (along with tendons and ligaments) that enable us to move.

Aside from helping us move more effectively from A to B, there are other added benefits to having muscle and increasing muscle mass. Now, I know the phrase 'muscle mass' sounds like it should be part of a scary looking protein powder commercial, but it's a good thing for both women and men. Aesthetically, muscles look great. They create strong curves and beautiful shapes and I can assure you that at least 98 per cent of the men and women that you associate with the hashtag #bodygoals will train in a way that helps them to develop and preserve muscle mass.

How to sculpt and grow your muscles

Bear with me as I get all sciencey for a moment – I really feel that getting a technical view of muscle growth will help you become realistic about achieving goals.

A lot of people (women in particular) are misled by advertising that suggests that all it takes to develop the body of a fitness model are a few Pilates classes and a vegan diet. While that may work for some of the genetically blessed, those beautiful fitness models (male and female) that you see dominating Instagram have all had to apply the following principles to their training regime in order to develop the muscle, and consequently the body, that they now have. In addition to food, hydration, sleep and rest, there are three major factors that contribute to the growth of your muscle:

1. Mechanical tension

Mechanical tension refers to big lifting, which is basically when you lift a weight that makes you feel like you have to channel your inner X-Man/Woman to even move it an inch. Placing adequate/heavy tension (load) on a muscle that is both stretched (bottom of a dead lift) or contracted (top of a dead lift) facilitates muscle growth[5]. Mechanical tension was absolutely one of the best and most life-changing aspects of my training programme as it really made a difference to the shape and composition of my body through increased muscle mass.

If you're still feeling scared about the notion of muscle growth, pretty please read my note on hypertrophy (see page 32). 'Heavy' is a relative concept, so 15kg to some may be monstrous, while to others it's just a warm-up weight – this is why this principle will greatly depend upon how much you have lifted in the past, and what heavy actually is to your body.

Even though it is a big part of muscle growth, I am not going to prescribe extremely heavy lifts within this book. Not because I don't want you to do them, but because with heavy lifts comes a greater risk of injury. I firmly believe that you should be training with a qualified strength coach before attempting to lift double your body weight. Luckily, mechanical tension is not the only mechanism through which we can facilitate muscle growth. Let's look at the other two.

2. Muscle damage

Did you know that when you train a muscle you actually damage it? My dad told me this when I was about 10 years old and competing heavily in gymnastics – I was complaining about some muscle soreness and he explained that it was because the excessive training had caused damage to the muscle. I was like, Waaaah? How is it possible that damage causes strength? It's actually a survival mechanism: create the damage and the body repairs it, but this time with an added layer of support (in this case, more muscle). How awesome is that?! Your human body is incredible! Muscle damage usually occurs when we do something out of the norm (think callisthenics), stretch a muscle while it's activated (think ashtanga yoga) and, last but not least, emphasise eccentric stress (e.g. slowly lowering out of a chin-up or into a squat). [6]

While a little muscle soreness is an important factor in achieving results, I don't want you to think that you should be crippled after every workout. All those memes of paralysed puppies on Instagram with the heading 'LEG DAY', although cute, are misleading and over-glorify the concept of muscle damage. Overtrain your muscles and you reduce the rate of recovery, which will just stop you from taking on the rest of your planned workouts. After my workouts you will feel sore, but not crippled.

3. Metabolic stress

This is probably the most commonly practised aspect of muscle growth because it has been made famous by bodybuilders who, let's face it, are undoubtedly the best at growing muscle. However, Google the prima ballerina Misty Copeland and look at her incredibly strong, muscular and yet feminine body. You'll quickly see that growing muscles isn't just a bodybuilder thing. Metabolic stress is also known as your higher rep, lower rest period training. It has been shown to make the most effective hormonal changes to induce muscle growth (and also fat loss – which is that whole 'tone' thing us ladies are always referring to).

The Vertue Method workouts within this book encompass the latter two of these mechanisms – in particular metabolic stress, because it also accommodates for effective fat loss too.

Glutes – the muscles that make you a better person
I believe that the gluteal muscles deserve their own mini-section in the book. The gluteals are a family of (potentially) powerful muscles called gluteus maximus,

BOOTY TRUTHS
The gluteal muscles, or glutes, are a highly desired piece of equipment on most female (and male) bodies and not only are they highly desired, they are highly required. To explain what I mean by the heading here, I want to assure you that it actually has very little to do with how they look, and more to do with function. Not only do stronger glutes look good in jeans, they make you faster, support your lower back, prevent knee and hip injury, provide your movement with correct stability, and so much more.

gluteus medius and gluteus minimus, all located around the pelvis. They are responsible for the coordination and execution of over 10 different movements, so it's really, really important that they are strong and, even more so, activated.

Butt facts that you need to know to grow the booty that will bring everyone to the yard:

Use it or lose it – Spend more than half your day sitting down? Then your glutes might well disappear: glutes don't stick around if they are not being used. Other muscles like the quadriceps (thigh muscles) can take over where the glutes have given up. Long term, this is bad news for your knees and lower back.

Variety is the spice of the booty – Volume, intensity, high reps, low reps, heavy, isolated: the glutes respond best to a variety of training techniques. Just like a plant needs sunlight, water and soil nourishment to grow, the glutes just won't sculpt and grow unless they are challenged in varying ways. The Vertue Method plan covers so many different techniques to ensure the shaping and sculpting of a firm pair of glutes.

Not all glutes are made equal – Like so many things within the body, what works for me may not necessarily work for you. So if you're not responding to light isolated work, try heavy. If you've been lifting heavy for a while now, try to bring it back to isolation work to ensure you're actually hitting your glutes.

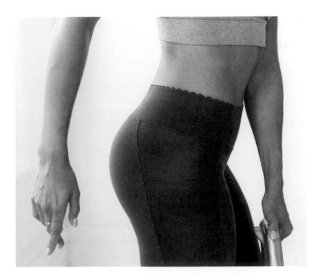

HOW TO LIFT

I want to eliminate the confusion, myths and mistakes that cloud the concept of 'lifting'. This section is by no means going to be directed at powerlifters wanting to hit PBs (personal bests) on their latest dead lift. I see weight training as something that will enhance your capability to move freely and so it's not so much geared towards massive and traditional strength gains (as that would be difficult without investing in some kind of squat rack). Instead it's directed at simplifying the most important and necessary lifts so that you can execute them with precision and grace (yes, I'm referring to both men and women here), and, most importantly, crush that fear of picking up something heavy in an effort to achieve a strong, firm and fantastic body.

In my opinion there are three key aspects to each lift:

1. The intention

The intention is essentially your mental state prior to entering the lift, and your level of concentration and focus. I believe these are crucial because the intention through which you move will ultimately lead to the outcome of the movement. Poor intention, lacking in focus and concentration, will eventuate in poor lifts, poor results and potential injury. Perfect intention, however, will bring about the elegant beast in you and enable the desired results.

Training in an environment that rivals the volume and lighting of an Ibiza superclub to me is not conducive to a concentrated intention. It's just going to distract you. A little music is fine to excite you for a slightly more intense workout, but you should still be able to devote your attention to the movement and practice. Before you enter each lift, think about the muscles you want to activate and give thought to the alignment cues for each exercise.

2. The alignment

The importance of alignment is obvious on paper, but seems to be the most neglected aspect of lifting. When that adrenaline and cortisol spike, the beat drops and you feel pumped to train, often the elegance and precision of movement flies out the window and our priority becomes going HARD or going HOME. Well, I'm here to remind you that going HARD without proper alignment means that you will go home, limping in pain, with a new injury that will need rehab and rest.

3. The breath

We can go without food for roughly seven days and water for a maximum of four days, but we can only live minutes without the breath. A smooth and efficient breath is key to the delivery of oxygen throughout the body; it can also help us to brace properly for a lift. In addition to this, as exemplified during yoga, the breath will help to maintain a calmer mind, as it has such a close relationship to the central nervous system (CNS).

Have you had to run for the bus with a head cold, unable to breathe properly? It's a really uncomfortable feeling, and yet we very often forget to breathe during exercise, not because we can't, but because we are focused on something else and we fall into irregular breathing patterns. The problem with irregular and unconscious breathing patterns is that if we are highly stressed, the way we breathe changes and becomes short, sharp and shallow. Learning to breathe with your movement not only helps you to be aerobically fitter, but also sends you into a sort of moving meditation. Yes, you can meditate while you squat.

EXERCISE SELECTION

There are hundreds – no, thousands – of complex exercises on the Internet, all promising incredible activation and isolation to 'sculpt and tone' the body.

I've seen fitness 'gurus' with feet in TRX straps and elbows on a BOSU (see the Glossary on page 263 for more on these) training their 'deep core', promising a thinner waist. Those of us who have ever had to watch daytime TV will have seen the seven-minute ab workout (or is it six?), with funky contraptions and promising 'more results in half the time'. Yet the best exercises tend to be the ones that have stood the test of time: think the squat, the lunge, the dead lift, pushing, pulling and twisting – these movements get the best results and are actually useful for us as humans to perform and perfect.

The majority of the exercises within my programme are compound movements. This means that they require multiple joints to move a resistance or weight. Because they move more than one joint, they demand more energy and are more taxing on the body (think more energy required, more calories burned, more efficient workout). In addition to this, compound movements simulate the same actions required in daily life. They are often termed as functional movements, and when mastered without dysfunction can help to minimise the risk of degenerative injuries further down the line. They also happen to sculpt and build a sexy body – male or female. By using weighted compound movements we will be strong, phat (pretty hot and tempting) and functional.

The key movements/exercises within the Vertue Method programme are: squat, dead lift, lunge, glute bridge, horizontal push, horizontal pull, vertical pull and vertical push.

All these exercises will have slight variations, but fundamentally this is what we're working with. By incorporating all these exercises and movements we balance the anterior, posterior and lateral aspects (front, back and sides) of the body to chisel, shape and mould a beautifully symmetrical physique. Moving through all planes of motion ensures that we don't just look amazing, we can actually DO amazing things too. There's nothing worse than beauty without function (that's just my opinion, but don't you agree?). I would much rather be Wonder Woman than Jessica Rabbit.

IT'S TIME TO LIFT

When you begin the programme, it is imperative that you read each description carefully, understanding the key alignment cues, before starting to lift. Even if you've been a keen lifter for a while, I urge you to refresh your skills and knowledge on the biomechanics of these highly effective but technical lifts.

For those of you who have never lifted weights before, the workout section is going to be somewhat confronting. However, I imagine that you're reading this because you want to be challenged.

LADIES: HYPERTROPHY IS NOT A DIRTY WORD!

Hypertrophy is defined as 'the enlargement of an organ or tissue from the increase in size of its cells'. When I speak of hypertrophy I am referring to the growth of muscle tissue and, ultimately, the growth – and therefore definition – of your muscles. Often we throw out the baby with the bathwater by avoiding weights and the concept of growing muscle completely. We do this just because we associate it with getting big or bulky or looking like Thor but with a smaller head.

Remember that the benefits of lifting far surpass that of just 'being able to lift heavy things'. You can build a sexy shape, improve your mental and physical health, and really, above all, you can cultivate a very strong sense of independence and power that is both motivating and satisfying. As soon as you begin to welcome it into your life you will experience just how good your body is supposed to feel.

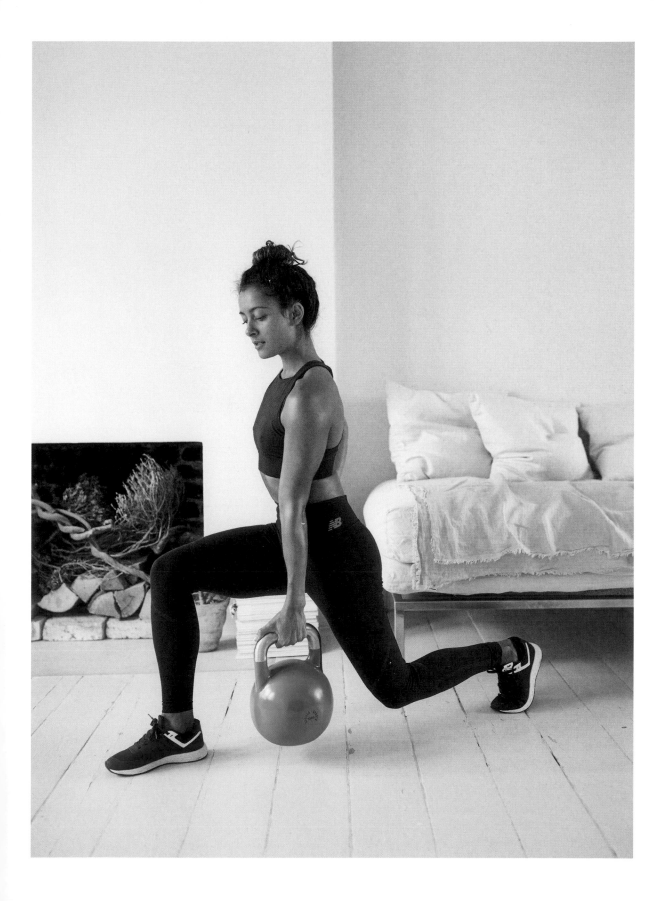

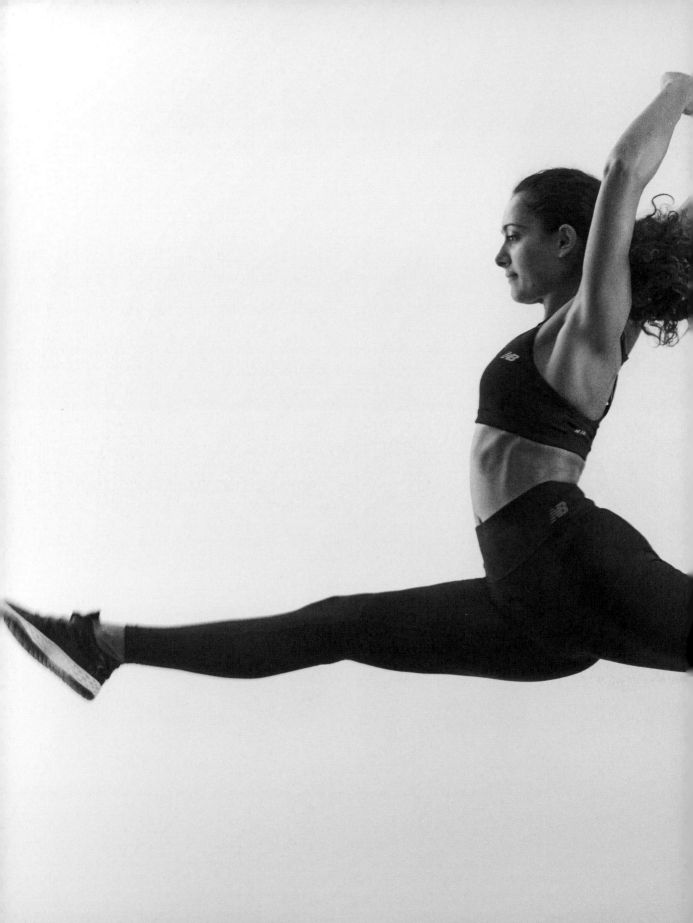

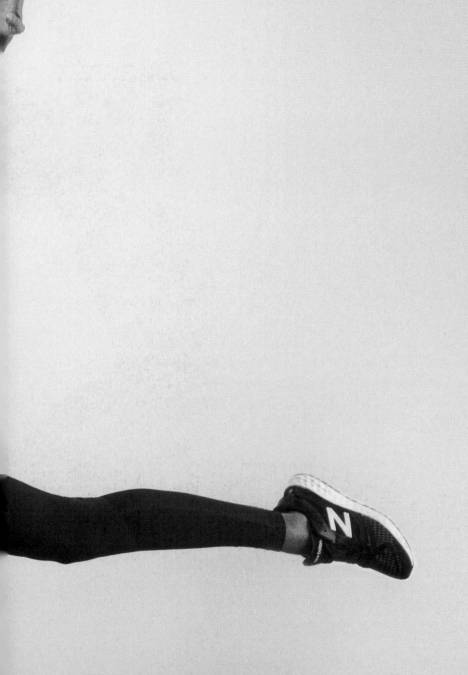

LENGTHEN

LENGTHEN

WHY LENGTHEN?

Hopefully you're reading this book because you understand the value of feeling good as well as looking good. Hopefully you understand that the Vertue Method body, while it loves to be lean and sculpted for aesthetic purposes, places the utmost worth on feeling really, really capable, because it knows that this is the best way to stay motivated for life, not just for the summer holidays. Well, that brings me to the topic of flexibility and mobility – the most underrated aspect of a fitness journey.

Let me first clarify what I meant when I named the pillar 'Lengthen'. I'm actually referring to posture and poise more than I am to the flexibility of individual muscles (but of course we will work on that too). I want you to be lengthened and tall in your stature because it's good not just for healthy biomechanics, but also for morale and mood. I also really believe that you're only as healthy as your joints are functionally mobile and, unfortunately, it's one of the areas that people tend not to pay enough attention to until they're injured or sick. So let's be smart and address this now.

The movement of your body from A to B is only possible because of your joints. If the movement of a joint is compromised, your ability to move is also compromised. Here's the really special part: your body is really nice; it tries to compensate so that you can continue to do the things that you want to (like work to earn a living to go on holidays and do fun stuff). However, the compensation doesn't always lead to the best outcome or to efficient biomechanics.

Yeah? So what? That doesn't stop me from achieving 'gainz' or getting my bikini body... Or does it?

Well, let's say that you take this beautiful body of yours to the gym with poor biomechanics and dysfunctional movement patterns. You decide to put it under load (lift weight) or do a cardio class that expects you to run, jump, twist, push and pull – also known as 'moving'. Well, soon enough you'll develop an ache (that's the body asking for help), then a twinge (that's the body yelling at you for help), then an injury (that's the body saying 'well, now we're both f**ked').

Suddenly your ability to train and move is hindered and you need to take time off. Hopefully it's just time out of the gym, but if it's bad enough, it will be off work too.

Now, the intention for this rant is not to scare you, but more to enliven a sense of value in feeling good and moving well; most people have no idea how good their body is supposed to feel.

Being a gymnast meant that I grew up around constant flexibility and mobility practices. When I began lifting weight (some 10 years later), I started to experience the frustration of not being able to perform a full-range squat, touch my toes or drop an outrageously large move on the dance floor without injury. It wasn't until I realised how little I was capable of in my body (compared to when I was a gymnast and dancer) that I decided to prioritise flexibility again. As soon as I began stretching and massaging regularly I remembered how good it felt to be mobile and free.

In addition to this, I have worked with many clients who are limited in movement – and they have expressed to me that gaining it back was one of the best feelings on the path to health and fitness.

There are three key aspects of the Lengthen pillar of my programme: flexibility, mobility and good posture.

WHAT IS FLEXIBILITY?

Flexibility is often defined as 'the quality of bending without breaking', yet it is much more complicated than just simply your ability to touch your toes. Anatomically speaking, flexibility refers to the length to which a muscle group can be stretched, whereas mobility refers to the range of motion of a particular joint. Rather interestingly, however, flexibility is a tricky one to understand. You would think that if you stretched a muscle, you would get more flexible, but the research shows that it's not that simple.

I often say that you're only as flexible as your nervous system is willing to let you be. One of the major reasons your nervous system may not allow that kind of flexibility is if there is a physiological issue preventing you from going into that range or depth of stretch. For example, if you have an injury, the nervous system is in charge of ensuring that you don't exacerbate that injury further. One of its protective mechanisms is to limit your range of motion to stop you from moving further than you should while healing an injury.

The nervous system isn't just in charge of damage control. Self-preservation and injury prevention are high on the list too: muscle or joint weakness is seen by the nervous system as a risk. In order to prevent you from injuring yourself, it will again limit range of motion to stop you from overextending beyond your capability. This is why I am always harping on to yogis about developing strength as a means to increase safe flexibility within the body.

Flexibility is a question of frequency, not intensity. If you spend all day at a desk, your body will actually mould itself to that shape, i.e. short hamstrings. You could come home and do an hour of intense hamstring stretching and it wouldn't make a difference because your body just spent nine hours sitting on a chair. So although you will be doing stretch sessions weekly, I also want you to think outside the desk. Could you use a standing desk? Could you take short but frequent walks throughout the day? The human body was not designed to be stuck behind a computer for 40 per cent of the day; it was designed for movement, jumping, sprinting, catching and Mick Jagger-style dancing.

Flexibility work, like training, must be structured and consistent – it really does require patience and, above all, it is imperative that you enjoy the process. The difference between hating a stretch routine and hating a workout routine is that many of us will put up with a workout routine purely for its aesthetic benefits. Yet sadly, because stretching doesn't yield those same 'visual' rewards we will be quick to skip it if we don't get any joy from it. Also, if we hate the process of stretching, chances are our nervous system will not be 'primed' for the release. Have you tried relaxing while doing something you hate? No, because it's impossible.

HAMSTRING HACK

On a weekly basis I am inundated with questions about tight hamstrings that just won't budge, and my answer is not as you might expect. For one, I don't reply with: 'Try stretching it.' This is because I'm sure many of you with chronically tight hamstrings have tried to stretch them. The other reason I don't say that is because very often hamstring tightness is caused by hamstring or adductor weakness – so a lot of the time my advice is to work on strengthening them. I know it sounds crazy and counterintuitive, but it's true. Support the structure with proper strength training and your nervous system will feel better about providing you with hamstring freedom.

The Vertue Method flexibility practices teach you how to enjoy the process. (I should also mention that it's a kind of love/hate thing – when you drop down into a glute stretch for the first time, chances are you'll be able to list a hundred different activities that you'd rather be doing, but the feeling of relief that comes from releasing tight hips far surpasses the discomfort of being within it.)

As I mentioned earlier, when I created the Vertue Method concept I had the time-poor in mind. As much as I wish I could get you to dedicate a full hour a day to stretching, it's just not realistic; ain't nobody got time for that. To accommodate for a lack of time, I have included some shorter flexibility sequences at night and a little yoga in every warm up.

WHAT IS MOBILITY?

Mobility refers to the range of motion within a specific joint. Different joints have different movement capabilities so, for example, open hips don't result in flexible shoulders as well. Each joint is surrounded by different muscles and therefore they require different types of stretches. Furthermore, just because someone can do the front splits does not automatically mean that they will be able to do the side splits – so both mobility and even flexibility are also movement specific, not just joint specific. Unlike stretching, where notable increases take a little while, the benefits of mobilising a joint through various techniques can be felt almost instantly.

Knot happy

Most of you will have heard of the term 'knot', and if you've ever had a massage you will have experienced the pain associated with knots. Think of your muscles as a collection of tiny ropes. Overuse of these ropes often leads to the development of a knot. These knots, or 'trigger points', can restrict movement and blood flow, eventually leading to further pain and dysfunctional movement patterns.

The pain from these trigger points can be both local and also referred (felt elsewhere within the body). If you're not sure what I'm talking about, ask your friend to squeeze the top of your shoulders (also known as the trapezius); very often the pain will spread right up into the head, even behind the eye. Or put an elbow in your gluteus medius (a true friend will always be willing to get close to your butt like that); you may feel a strong pain in the butt, but it may also refer downwards into the leg, or into your back. Very often when you have this knot-like tension within the body, you will feel as though you want to stretch it out. However, imagine trying to release a knot from a rope by stretching and pulling at its two ends. It certainly won't unravel it and, in fact, it could exacerbate it further. This means that you cannot outstretch tension. Even the most flexible person you know will have these trigger points around the body, and they can't be stretched into freedom.

Through a series of weekly self-myofascial and trigger point release sessions (kind of like giving yourself a massage), you will very soon realise how delicious movement is supposed to feel. These practices will improve your capability to move through workouts by having the mobility to sit deeper in your squats, lunges and dead lifts, facilitating better potential for hypertrophy as well as helping you to live in a pain-free body.

WHAT IS GOOD POSTURE?

My old martial arts teacher used to tell me that good posture is when your body is in harmony with the force of gravity. How many of us actually consider that concept when we are typing away at our computers or waiting in line to buy our groceries?

Not many. It doesn't really cross our minds. In fact most of us think of good posture as sitting up tall because our elders told us to do so. We rarely give it thought, until, of course, pain and suffering rear their ugly heads and the physiotherapist or osteopath remind us that our spine is out of alignment, causing us this pain.

Spinal alignment

Do you know the purpose of the curves in your spine? The S shape enables the body to withstand different kinds of force, almost like a shock absorber. If the spine was straight up and down, we would simply not be able to

KEY BENEFITS OF STRETCHING AND MOBILISING

Injury prevention

I always feel as though people don't really care about injury until it's too late. Being able to move more freely will prevent your body from pulling a muscle or ligament.

Better posture

Spending a lot of time in one position can cause the joints to fuse in a certain position. This makes it hard to stand/sit with good posture even if you want to.

Improved circulation

If a muscle is in spasm its blood supply is restricted; by helping to release these trigger points you can improve blood circulation.

Improved libido (and potentially better sex)

While there isn't any scientific data to back this up, it kind of goes without saying that if you improve your ability to move freely and circulate blood through the body (especially to the genitals) you may very well support performance and therefore excitement between the sheets. I have had many men and women discuss improvements to their sexual experiences through an increase in mobility and flexibility.

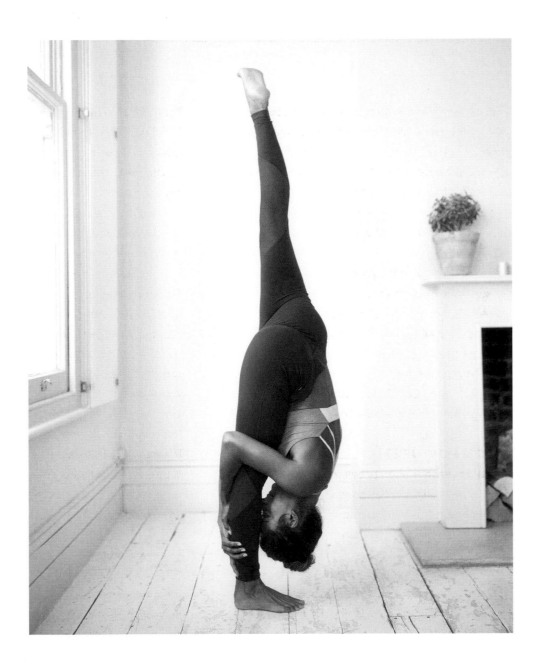

move in the way that we do. Importantly, the spine also houses the spinal cord, which is a key part of our central nervous system. So, considering all this, maintaining the health of your spine is important. Another key reason for the health and alignment of our spine, pelvis and ribcage is that it affects the positioning, and therefore potentially the function, of some pretty essential equipment like the heart and the digestive and reproductive organs. Sometimes just minor discrepancies in our structural balance and alignment can cause visceral functioning issues.

HEALTHY AND UNHEALTHY POSTURE

Hyperkyphosis

The upper spine has a natural C-shaped curve, but over time the curves within the spine can become exaggerated. While hyperkyphosis can be caused by a deformity that occurs in the womb, it can also come from constant unconscious movement patterns in response to lifestyle habits. Does this posture remind you of how you scroll through Instagram?

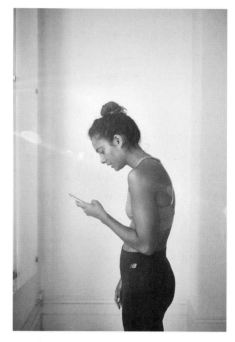

Hyperlordosis

Lumbar hyperlordosis is actually quite common. It is a position where the natural curve of the lumbar region of the back is slightly or dramatically accentuated. Often this posture is also associated with 'flaring ribs'. A flaring ribcage can cause major middle back pain as well as shoulder, neck and headache tension. I also like to call this posture the 'high-heel, night-out, shake-what-yo-Mumma-gave-you' posture – it can very often be deemed sexy, but my goodness have I seen it cause a lot of pain (in my body and the bodies of my clients). There are a number of causes, including tight hip flexors, weak lower abs, weak glutes and sometimes just poor postural awareness.

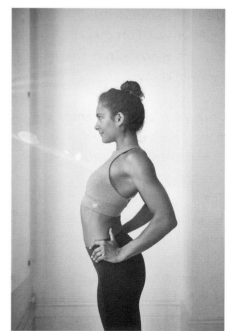

Balanced

Perfect posture is almost indefinable, because we all have very differently built bodies. However, there are a few cues that can help you to find a healthier stature.

Firstly it's imperative that there is a natural curvature of the spine as well as correct ribcage alignment. Too much extension (hyperlordosis) is just as bad as too much flexion (hyperkyphosis) as it inhibits the diaphragm's ability to contract and relax, ultimately affecting your breathing patterns. This can then result in neck and upper chest breathing, which can place increased stress on the nervous system.

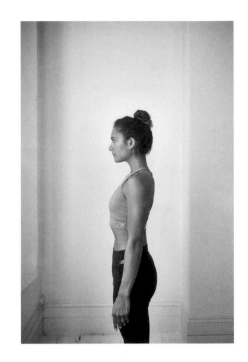

Stand with the back of your head against the corner of a wall. I say the corner here so that if you are blessed with a booty, you can still allow your tail bone to touch the wall. You will do this by enabling the wall to slide in between your butt cheeks – look, it's not the most elegant description but I assure you it will be helpful for those of you with booty.

Place your feet hip distance apart. Your tail bone and mid thoracic spine (the spine in between the shoulder blades) should be against the wall.

There should be less than 5cm between your neck and lower back against the wall. A larger gap could indicate poor postural habits or structure.

To correct it, try taking a deep exhalation, allowing the ribcage to pull inward as you keep the chin tucked in and head against the wall. At the same time, think about aiming to get your imaginary 'belt buckle' towards your breastbone.

MOBILITY SEQUENCE

This sequence will help you find the knots within the body
that are preventing you from moving efficiently. You're going
to press into some of the hard tissue that forms in and around
the knots using a mobility ball. It's going to hit some sore
points, but persist – to increase flexibility you need to release
tightness. Take a minimum of five breaths for each body part.

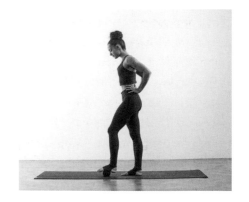

Feet
Place one foot on a tennis or mobility ball and apply a firm
pressure. Roll the foot forwards and backwards over the ball,
holding over areas of tension.

Gluteus medius and piriformis
From a seated position, place your feet flat on the floor, hip
distance apart. Put your hands on the floor behind you for
support. Lift the hips and place the ball at the gluteus medius
or the piriformis (as pictured). Put your left foot on top of
your right knee. Use your hands and feet to control how much
weight you apply on the ball. Roll the ball from the inside to
the outside of the glute.

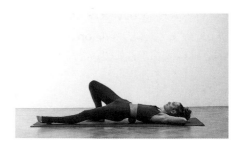

Erectors
Lie on your back and lift it slightly so that you can place the
ball under it (as pictured). Keep one knee bent so that you
can take some of the pressure of your body in the leg, rather
than putting all of it into the ball. Rather than rolling over the
ball, let yourself place pressure on the tight and painful areas,
moving the ball with your hand to change pressure points.

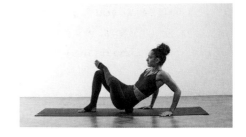

Rhomboids
Place the ball on the floor and move your back onto it, allowing
the ball to sit on the muscle in between the shoulder blades.
Keep the knees bent to maintain stability, and gently rock your
body up and down over the ball.

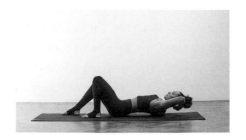

Infraspinatus

It's best to find this trigger point from a seated position. Sit up and use your left arm to reach around to grab hold of your right shoulder. Run your fingertips along the scapula spine (the first bony part that you can feel sticking out of your shoulder blade). The ball will be placed right under this spot. Grab the ball and place it under the scapula spine, slowly coming to lie down on your side, so that your body ends up on top of the ball. Gently rock up and down to find the tension.

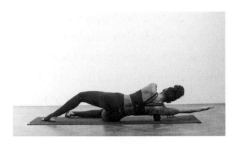

Levator scapulae

Standing close to a wall, place the ball on the levator scapulae (as pictured). Move your body up against the wall and use your legs to press your levator scapulae into the wall. Roll up and down without rolling on the spine.

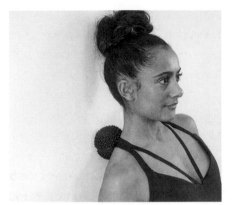

Trapezius

Standing close to a wall, place the ball on the trapezius (as pictured). Move your body up against the wall (you will need to be slightly side on and use your legs to press your trapezius into the wall). Gently roll along the trapezius.

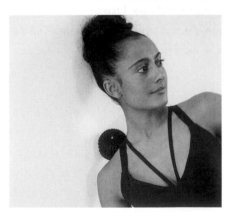

Pectoralis minor

Place the ball on the chest, close to the shoulder. Place the palms over the ball with your elbows bent out to the side. Inhale here, and as you exhale apply pressure to the ball – moving your elbows up and down to create gentle movement in the ball.

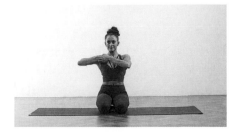

FLEXIBILITY SEQUENCE

This yoga-inspired sequence is mostly aimed at releasing built-up tension in the hips because the majority of your movement stems from there. By releasing the tightness in your pelvic region, legs and lower back you facilitate freer movement and you will be able to move deeply through each workout exercise, so when you hit your deepest squat, you will activate more muscle fibres than if you were to take a modest curtsy. More muscle recruited, more energy required, more energy burned. Take some time out of your evening to go through each of these postures, staying in each for 10 breaths. Inhale deeply, exhale completely. Not only will the slow breathing help your muscles relax, you will also prepare the body for a better night's sleep. I don't believe that stretching should be painful; a mild stretching sensation will be enough to release the tightness.

Rag Doll
Stand with your feet hip width apart. Bend the knees and drop the body forward, letting your chest rest upon your thighs. Take hold of either elbow and relax the back of the neck.

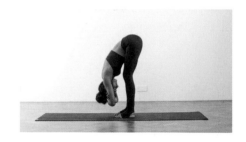

Kneeling Lunge
Come into a lunging position with your back knee on the floor. Sink the hips forward allowing your hands to support you either side of the front leg.

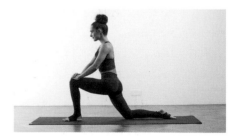

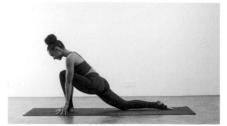

Half Splits Pose

From the Kneeling Lunge position, shift your hips backwards so that the front leg becomes straight and the back leg becomes bent. Move your hands back slightly to support you and round your spine so that your body drops forward. Relax the back of the neck.

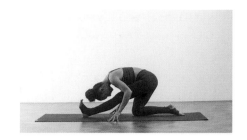

Lizard with Backfoot Grab

Move forward back into the lunge, however this time both your hands will be on the inside of your front leg. Bend the back leg and, if you can, grab the ankle with your opposite hand (so that you are twisting the upper body). Start to pull the heel in towards the buttocks. If you cannot reach the back leg, use a towel or yoga strap, hooking it around the back foot for more leverage. For a more advanced variation, bring the front elbow to the floor.

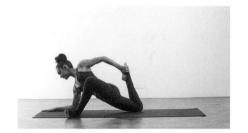

Pigeon

Come back into a lunge position. Lift your front ankle and place the knee down to the floor. Move the front knee out to the side slightly so that it is pointing to the top corner of your mat. Try to keep the hips square as you let your body come down to the floor, resting your forehead on your forearms or all the way down to the floor. If you feel as though your hips are falling to one side, place a block or folded cushion under your hips to keep them lifted and centred.

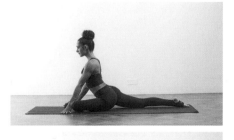

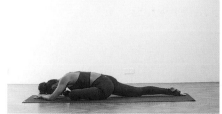

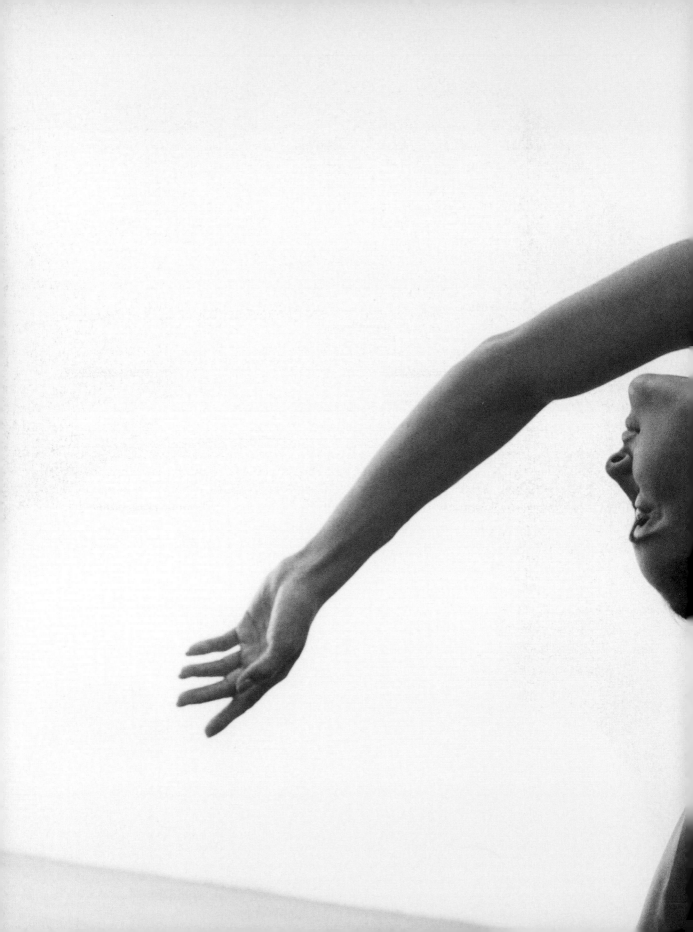

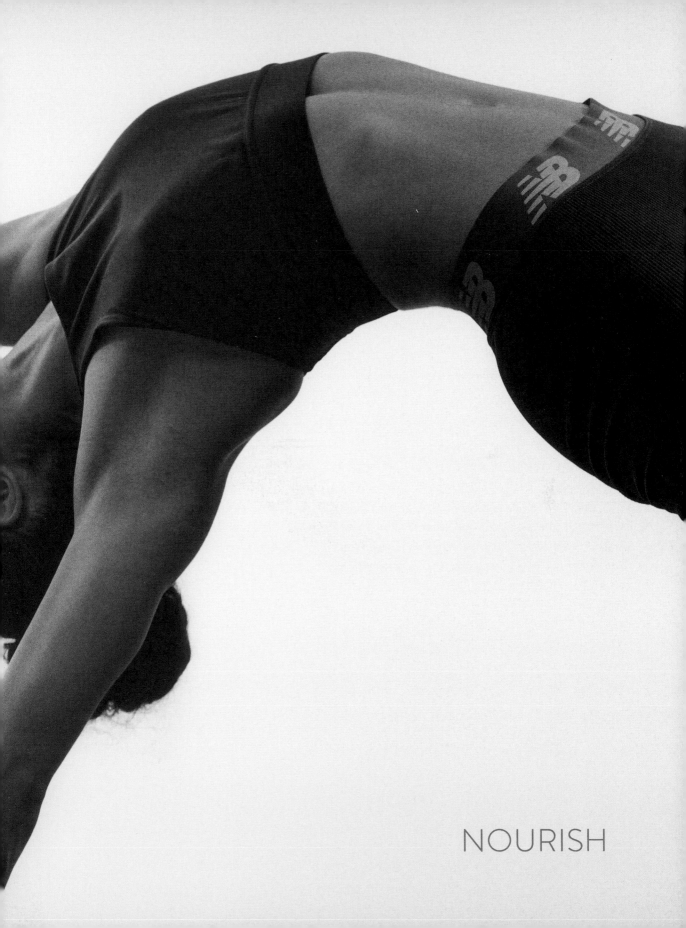

NOURISH

NOURISH

WHY NOURISH?

To really nourish ourselves I believe we need to feed both our bodies and our minds. The Nourish pillar is divided into two categories: dietary nourishment (for the body) and mental nourishment (via meditation, for the mind). And in fact, when you meditate you support your body and when you eat well you support your mind, so the two things are deeply and intrinsically linked.

Before I tell you how to nourish yourself, as always I want to break down the why and a little of the science. I think that education creates the best motivation; when we understand the reason for doing something we are just way more likely to do it. For me, staying motivated to lift, lengthen, meditate and eat well is directly linked to knowing how and why it benefits me.

The word nourish is itself derived from the Latin verb *nutrire* – to nurture.

The truth is, I could write you the most perfect diet in the history of diets and, if you couldn't follow it, well, it wouldn't be so perfect would it? Likewise, demanding that you dedicate an hour a day to sitting cross-legged on the floor for meditation practice, when you find it uncomfortable to sit for even one minute in a chair, isn't going to help you unlock the joy-enhancing powers of meditation – it will just make you dislike meditation and probably make you dislike me too.

What I will provide for you within this pillar is what I believe to be the most important aspects of feeling truly wholesome, not just skinny or lean. Let's learn to nurture our bodies into health and into an improved life experience.

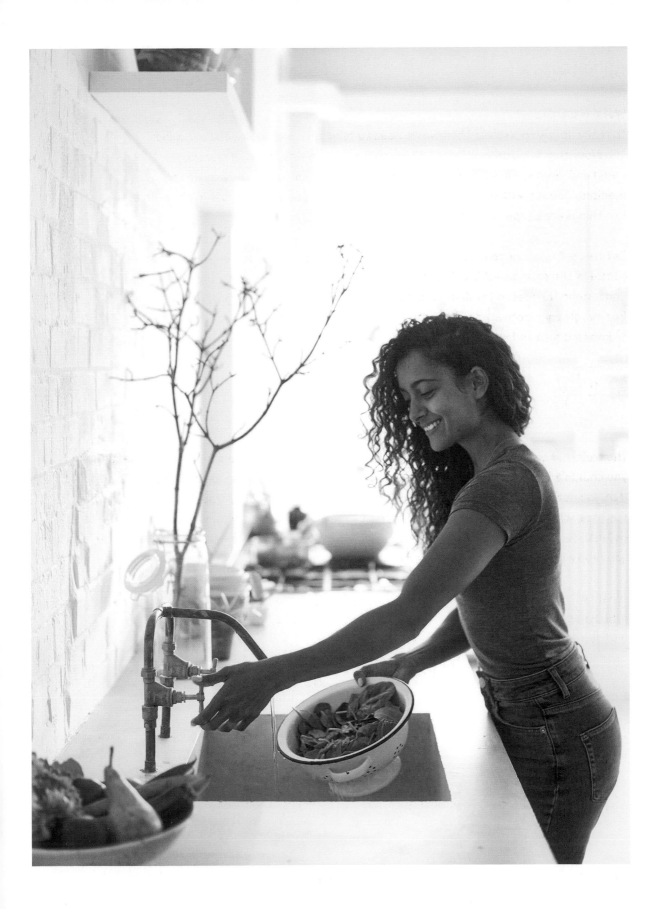

PART ONE: DIET

WHAT IS IT?

The word diet itself refers simply to the foods eaten by a particular person (or group). However, because 'dieting' is so widespread, the notion of a diet is now based more around calorie or food group restriction.

The bottom line is that quick, intense and short-term 'diets' don't work; they may cause weight loss temporarily, but what is the point in that apart from making you feel bad when the weight comes back on? If you are currently overweight, underweight, feeling low in energy, lethargic, experiencing digestive issues, etc., then the chances are you may well require a change to your diet – that is, a change to the foods you consume in order to nourish yourself into wellness. A diet shouldn't be considered a short-term solution, rather an evolution into a better way of living.

STRONG, FIT AND LEAN BODY FORMULA

Nothing I'm going to say here is revolutionary – it's all out there on the World Wide Web. I'm just going to condense it and make it easier to digest (excuse the pun).

If you want to lose weight you need to consume less food than your body burns for energy each day. If you want to gain weight, you need to consume more food than your body burns each day. Simple, right? Not exactly. This concept has been around for many decades, and yet still many of us find it quite difficult to lose fat and maintain or build muscle. I believe that this is because there is a little more to achieving and, more importantly, keeping the body you want.

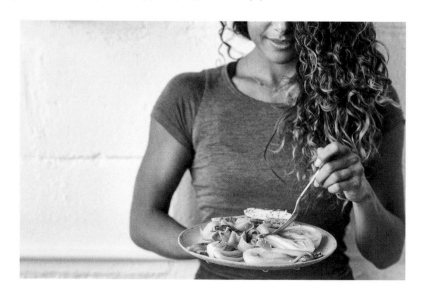

The Vertue Method philosophy includes the following principles:

1. Positive intention
Learning to love and value yourself even before you've seen results.

2. Balancing energy expenditure
Calories in vs. calories out.

3. Consuming the nutrients that the body needs to function like a boss
Balancing macro- and micronutrients.

4. Adequate hydration
Often the most neglected aspect of looking leaner and feeling more energised.

5. Intuition
Information is not knowledge; only YOU know your body.

Notice how I didn't mention alkalising or drinking seven bottles of lemon juice a day, or restricting red apples because they have more sugar than green apples... No. Because you can have the body you want without having to resort to drastic dieting measures. While those diets often promise and can deliver quick results, the extreme nature of them is impossible to maintain, not just physically but psychologically too. Willpower is not an everlasting pool of strength; in fact, many scientists and psychologists liken it to a muscle that can be fatigued with overuse.

This book is about developing balance, not sucker-punching the body from one extreme to the next. Let's now look at those principles in a little more detail.

1. POSITIVE INTENTION

Ah, here we are again, back at intention. If you have been paying attention you will have noticed that this is something I address in the lifting section too. Intention is the seed of everything that manifests in our life and thus will determine the action and the outcome through which it occurs. Dieting with the intention of getting skinny quickly is very different to dieting with the intention of getting healthy for life. While both relate to a change of diet, the type of action taken to achieve the desired effect will be very, very different. I'm sure I don't have to tell you that one of them is going to be a painful process and the other much more enjoyable.

So, before you embark on your fitness/health goal I believe that you must first ask yourself why it is that you want it. Why are you here? Why do you believe you need to change? This kind of information will ultimately shape your food choices.

Eating because you want to become stronger and more energised is far more encouraging than eating to fit the ever-changing social standards of what it is to be sexy. I also think shifting your perspective from eating to become thinner (which in itself sounds a little contradictory) to eating to feel like an optimally functioning human, means that you will reap the benefits of both – you will feel great and, if it's healthy for you to do so, you will lose body fat.

Allowing your intention to incorporate self-love and self-respect is an important part of achieving your health goals, because – contrary to popular belief – we are more motivated by love than hate. Too many nights spent on social media scrolling through pictures of men and women whose bodies you envy can cultivate a sort of self-loathing. It's an empty feeling that we mistakenly believe can only be healed when we have 'what they have', when we 'eat clean' or diet harder. But because the intention is steeped in a sense of self-dissatisfaction, the exercise and healthy eating tend to come from a place of punishment – punishing ourselves for not living up to our own expectations. The good news is that punishment is not an effective form of motivation; reward and pleasure are.

Who would have thought it, huh? So your intention has to reflect love, joy, pleasure, nourishment, nurturing and happiness – you know, the good shit. The Vertue Method plan is going to help you reset the dial towards all those things.

2. BALANCING ENERGY EXPENDITURE (CALORIES IN VS. CALORIES OUT)

I don't count calories, but I am very aware of the calorific energy requirements of my body, especially how many calories I require to stay alive and remain strong, lean and healthy. Understanding your calorific requirements is going to help you achieve results and get the most from your diet. However, becoming obsessive about numbers is just going to lead to disordered eating and yo-yo dieting. Let's start with some basic science.

What is a calorie?

Some people act as if 'calorie' is the name for a scary monster living in the fridge eagerly waiting to seduce you into fat gain, but it is in fact just the name for a unit of energy. To very quickly explain:

A calorie is simply a reference to the energy potential of a particular food.

When we chow down on that delicious bowl of pasta, we're essentially putting energy into our body that our body will use up in an effort to keep us alive. The quality of your food choices can obviously affect the quality of your life (when I say life, I'm referring to the act of being alive, brain function, energy levels, metabolism, etc.).

Your food is your fuel, and that is a very important way to think about it because it should put a stop to any fearmongering around food groups caused by the media or even created within your own mind. Unfortunately, we can't get around the evidence-based notion/law of energy expenditure: losing weight requires a calorie deficit and putting on weight requires a surplus.

However, not all calories affect the body in the same way. There are roughly 67 calories in a serving of oatmeal cookies. There are also roughly 67 calories in 440g of lettuce. Does that make them equal? In energy potential yes, but what makes them not the same is obviously the quantity required to get the same energy potential. What also differentiates the cookies and the lettuce is the macro- and micronutrient breakdown, which is why not all food is equal in providing what is needed to reveal the inner Supreme Being in you. More of that coming up.

Learning to eat in accordance with your energy needs is healthy, not restrictive. If you've been eating at a surplus for a long time, and you do need to lose fat, it is important that you bring about balance by learning to eat at a healthy deficit to facilitate the fat loss, while ensuring that the underlying superhero muscle remains.

The set up of the 28-day reset plan eliminates the need to constantly count calories. For all the geeks (like me) I've included the various formulas to understanding your body's energy requirements at the back of this book (see page 262).

3. CONSUMING THE NUTRIENTS THAT THE BODY NEEDS TO FUNCTION LIKE A BOSS

This is a slightly bigger topic and is divided into two categories: macronutrients and micronutrients. Macronutrients are protein, carbs and fat, while micronutrients are vitamins and minerals. Let's start with the macronutrients:

Protein

The importance of protein far surpasses just building muscle. It kind of builds all the other good stuff too, like hair, skin, nails, cardiac muscle (the muscle that is the heart – yeah, so pretty important), bones, cartilage and even blood. Aside from structure, protein is also required for optimal functioning of the body and its organs, production of enzymes and antibodies, and even the transportation of other important atoms and molecules. So when someone says that the need for protein is a myth, tell him or her that until you're ready to live in the body of an extraterrestrial, energetic light being, you'll be sticking to protein.

We can store fat (in fat cells) and carbohydrates (as glycogen), but as our body has no way to store protein as an extra reserve somewhere, we need to eat it consistently.

When you eat food with protein, the body breaks it down into amino acids, and those amino acids are then rebuilt to make protein that the body can use to build, well, everything. So it's aminos that make protein consumption so important; they are the building blocks of the protein within our body. There are 20 amino acids in your body's proteins, and nine of them are essential to our diet, meaning that we as humans can't synthesise them through our own chemical reactions, we must get them from our diet. These amino acids have various different roles within the body, from brain function to literally building tissue. So it's incredibly important that we try to consume them all. A complete protein is one that contains all nine of these essential amino acids. Most animal protein sources are complete, but if you combine certain plant-based proteins like rice and beans, you can create a meal with a complete amino acid profile (yay for vegans!).

Vertueous protein sources

Protein is found in an abundance of foods, from animals to plants, and of course in protein supplements. The value of a protein is based on your ability to digest it and on its amino acid profile (the building blocks we were discussing above). So generally speaking we want to consume proteins that are easily digested within the body and that have a wonderful range of amino acids, especially the essential amino acid leucine that is particularly important for protein synthesis.

Protein quantities in food

The table overleaf is a basic guide to some of the more common protein sources available to you. These amounts are based on 100g servings, mostly cooked.

PLANT POWER

Here's the good news: plants have protein (and consequently amino acids) too, so it is possible to get enough protein in a less slaughter-y way if you want to (I don't judge the decision either way but I do believe it's really important to remember where meat comes from and try not to be disconnected from the truth of it). I'm not here to tell you to give up meat – that is a very personal choice – but I will say that vegetables are brilliant too, and cheaper, so regardless of whether you want to be vegan or vegetarian, don't rule out the concept of hitting your protein targets with vegetables. If you are going to go completely plant-based in protein, it's important to ensure that you're getting a wide range of them.

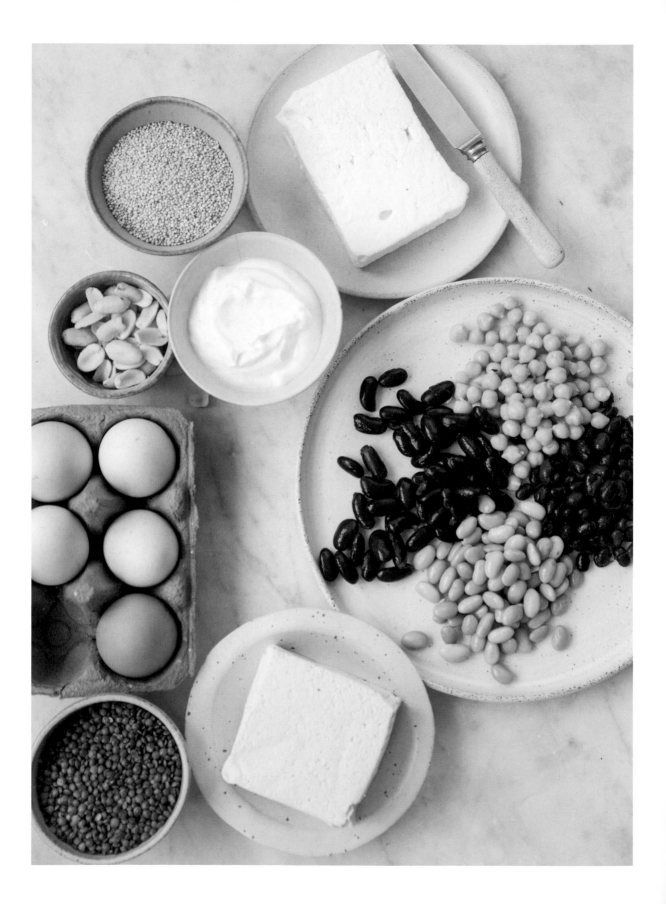

COMMON PROTEIN SOURCES

FOOD (100g cooked – as per method indicated – or raw where specified)	PROTEIN IN GRAMS	HOW MUCH SHOULD YOU EAT TO GET THE RECOMMENDED 20G PER MEAL?	NOTES
Kidney beans (boiled)	9g	200g	Very lean source of vegan protein with only 0.9g fat per 100g.
Soybeans and edamame (boiled)	12.4g	175g	Although soy has its opponents, it is high in protein and particularly in leucine (an important amino acid for vegans). This serving gives you 4.9g leucine, which is pretty awesome for a vegan source of protein.
Lentils (boiled)	9g	200g	Another very lean source of protein for vegans, which is great for not overshooting fat intake. Lentils are a great source of fibre, which we know keeps us regular (yes please). A high fibre intake has also been linked to reduced heart disease.
Tofu (fried)	17g	125g	Tofu is quite a controversial topic because soybeans are very often labelled as causing cancer and killing unicorns. Unfortunately 81 per cent of soybean crops are genetically modified organisms (GMOs), although almost all of that goes to feeding livestock. There are plenty of soy products like tofu and tempeh that are clearly labelled non-GMO. Men, if you're worried about the feminising effects of soy, it's just not true (see page 63).
Chickpeas (boiled)	9g	200g	The fibre and protein content of chickpeas makes them extremely satisfying; 200g of chickpeas also contains around 26 per cent of your RDI of iron.
Black beans (boiled)	8g	200g	Fibrous and delicious, these beans are a very lean source of protein. I also find them less irritating on the gut than lentils and chickpeas.

Quinoa (boiled)	4.4g	450g	Quinoa is a complete protein (it contains all nine essential amino acids). However, as you can see, you would need to eat a lot to get the 20g serving. My recommendation is to mix it with another, more protein-dense ingredient.
Egg (1 large raw)	6g	150g or 3 large eggs	Eggs are an awesome source of protein. Biotin, found in the yolk, helps to maintain the health of skin, hair and nails. It also supports the functioning of the nervous system. I urge you, for the sake of the hens and your health, to choose organic eggs.
Milk (whole)	3.2g	600ml	Milk is controversial because of the way it's often obtained. Without going into detail, some industrial dairy farms have practices that result in the inhumane treatment of animals, which also affects the quality of the milk itself. Organic dairy farms work differently, so it's worth buying organic where possible. The more we choose organic, the better the industry will get.
Feta cheese (raw)	14g	150g	Feta is made from goat's or sheep's milk or a combination. Goat's milk in particular contains less lactose than cow's which makes it easier to digest, particularly if you find yourself a little sensitive to lactose.
Greek yoghurt (raw)	10g	200g	Again, see my points on milk above. What is great about yoghurt, however, is the fact that it's fermented and contains probiotics, which are important for your gut flora. Gut bacteria does more than just support your digestive system; they even support immunity and help to produce vitamins too.
Mackerel (raw)	18.6g	100g or 1 fillet	A really great source of omega-3 fatty acids. As long as it's locally caught using traditional methods, mackerel is a sustainable fish.

Salmon (raw)	20g	100g	Salmon, though delicious, is overfished. I source farmed salmon, which I know is heavily debated because of questionable and unethical methods in certain fish farms, however there are some farms doing it correctly and sustainably. The New Zealand King Salmon Company and the Loch Duart farm in the UK are two examples of farms rearing their fish the right way. Essentially it's important to do your research before purchasing.
Haddock (grilled)	19.9g	100g or 1 small fillet	The great thing about haddock is that it tastes relatively mild so it's a good choice for those of you wanting to eat more fish but who don't like the taste. From a sustainability perspective it can be tricky to determine the origins of the fish, and some locations like the North East Atlantic are completely depleted of haddock species and should not be fished.
Chicken breast (cooked)	30g	65g or less than ½ breast	The quality of the chicken you purchase is important not just for animal rights, but also your health. Aim to avoid purchasing battery hens (and eggs), choosing free-range and organic as much as possible.
Turkey (roasted)	26g	80g	Turkey is rich in protein and low in fat. Contrary to popular belief, it does not make you sleepy from its L-tryptophan content, in fact it contains less than chicken.
Minced beef (baked)	24g	80g	Grass-fed beef is high in B vitamins, iron, selenium and other important vitamins and minerals. However, if the quality of your meat is poor, you really need to make sure you're getting more vegetables in the diet to make up for the lack in the meat. High-quality meat is usually very expensive, so if you're not able to afford it, eat less of it, or none at all.

What about protein supplements?

Personally, I love protein powder. Not because I think it's superior to a 'whole food', but because it saves me time and helps me to hit my protein targets.

As I have touched on, not all proteins were created equal. We need to look at their ability to be digested as well as their amino acid profiling, because those aspects will influence their effectiveness within your body.

Opposite is a table of some of the more popular protein supplements.

Not all proteins were created equal. We need to look at their ability to be digested as well as their amino acid profile to determine their effectiveness within your body.

How to choose the right protein supplement for you?

The answer is simple. I'm not going to focus on the general bioavailability (which refers to our body's ability to digest and absorb the nutrients) of a protein per se – I'm going to remind you to listen to YOUR body. While whey may have the highest bioavailability according to science, if you feel awful when you consume it, it's clearly not the best option for you. Eggs can also disagree with some people's guts, as can quinoa or pea protein. Age, genetics and lifestyle play a huge part in how we react to our foods, so pay attention to your symptoms. If you feel bloated after any foods, but especially protein, it's best to switch things up.

PROTEIN SUPPLEMENTS

PROTEIN	BENEFITS
Whey	Whey is a complete protein because it contains all nine essential amino acids. A study has also shown it to help lower appetite hormones in obese men[7] as well as increase fat-free mass when coupled with resistance training[8]. Hydrolysate protein is the best form of whey as it's extremely absorbable and tends to be a lot gentler on the gut.
Casein	Casein comes from cow's milk. It is a slow-digesting protein, and creates a gel-like consistency when mixed with liquid. The benefit of slow-digesting proteins is that consumption before bed can help to promote post-exercise overnight recovery.
Soy	Soy is a tricky one, as it has received a very confusing 'dual-reputation' for being a 'health' supplement, as well as being a 'harmful' supplement. There was speculation that the isoflavones in soy, that can have potentially oestrogenic effects, were going to 'feminise' men (think, the lowering of testosterone and the increase of man boobs, plus an amazing ability to multitask), but the scientific evidence has not confirmed that this is the case and soy has not been seen to feminise or lower the quality of sperm in men. In fact, there is some research to suggest that soy consumption may actually prevent breast cancer in post-menopausal women, as well as potentially lower cholesterol. Soy is also a complete protein.
Hemp	Hemp is a really interesting ingredient. It's not quite a complete protein, with the limiting amino acid being lysine, but it contains edestin and albumin, which have been shown to have some extremely positive effects on our immune systems. Edestin aids digestion, and hemp is the best for those with sensitive stomachs.
Pea and rice blend	The reason I have put these two together is that, like many celebrity couples, they are better as a pair. Rice protein is high in cysteine and methionine but low in lysine, whereas pea protein is low in cysteine and methionine but high in lysine. Together they make a complete protein with an amino acid profile that comes very close to whey.
Egg	Egg protein powder does not taste amazing and it smells like farts, at least the ones that I have tried. If I'm going to use egg for protein, I'd rather just put the egg whites straight into the smoothie as they have no taste. Egg protein is really well absorbed by the body, and is a complete protein.

A WORD ON VEGANISM

I am not a vegan, but as you will notice, throughout the book I express concerns for animal and environmental welfare, encouraging the reduction of animal product intake. I just want to clarify my reasons for this so that you have some understanding on where I am coming from.

In 2008 I tried veganism. I went cold turkey, meaning I woke up one morning and stopped all animal product consumption. I had very minimal nutritional knowledge and made no conscious effort to understand what a vegan would need to stay energised and healthy through a transition. I was passionate about eliminating my own contribution to the terrible practices that can occur in the name of meat and dairy production. Before giving up meat, I had followed a strict Paleo diet (which is probably the most animal-eating diet there is).

Proudly, I stuck to veganism for two years, but unfortunately I became excruciatingly ill. I developed severe anaemia, to the point where I had to stop teaching yoga due to chronic exhaustion. To cut a long story short, this sickness came about because I was uneducated about how to eat properly as a vegan. I didn't consume enough protein, and I didn't get a wide variety of fruit and vegetables – which can help to make up for the amino acids you might be missing with a smaller protein intake. I went to see a dietician, who advised me to start eating meat again to regain my health. The animal activist in me was sad about it, but my body was happy.

Needless to say, that experience of sickness scared me, but I know that it was purely my lack of education and organisation that got me into that position – not veganism itself. In fact, you can be perfectly healthy on a vegan diet if you are diligent with your macro- and micronutrient intake. I do not want my story of illness to turn you off the concept of reducing your meat intake; instead I hope that it serves as a reminder of the importance of eating a balanced diet.

Today, I am more mindful with my food choices. The nature of life on this planet is that we will never be completely 'cruelty-free', but we can all take a more loving approach to our life practices. In fact, for the sake of our children and the future of this planet, reducing your meat and dairy intake may not just be a compassionate choice, but a necessity.

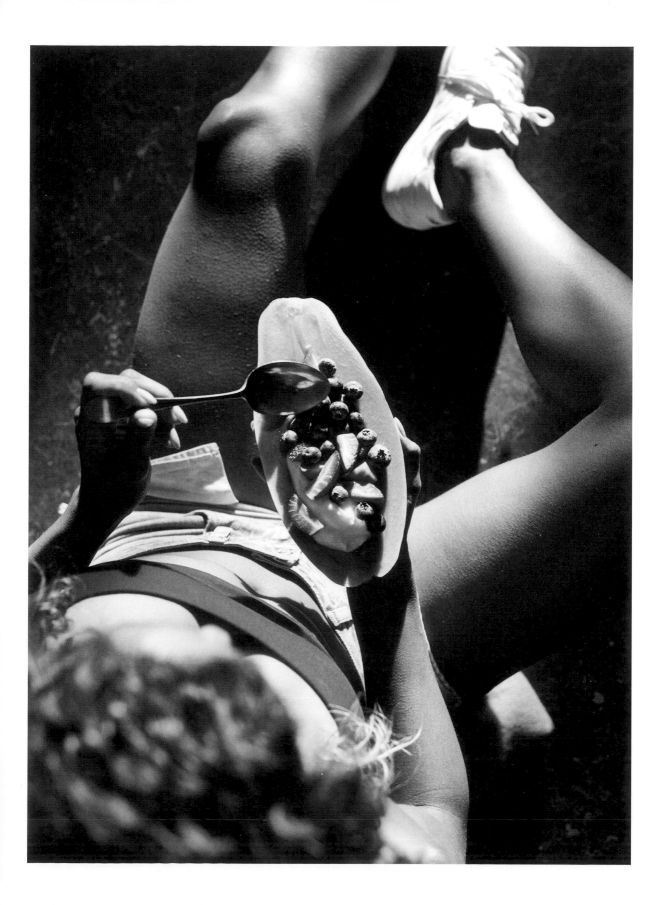

Carbohydrates

Poor carbies; I feel carbohydrates can be likened to Andy Dufresne in *The Shawshank Redemption* or Sirius Black in *Harry Potter* (wrongfully accused is what I'm going for, if you haven't seen those movies or read the books). Many diets out there promote the reduction or even complete elimination of carbohydrates, because apparently they are evil and will make you gain weight. So before we point the fat finger at carbohydrates, let's have a really quick look at what they are. Sometimes we are afraid of things because we fail to understand them, so I hope that in learning a bit more about carbohydrates you will feel less scared of consuming them.

Carbohydrates are classified by the complexity/length of their chemical structure in the form of saccharides (aka sugar). I'm going to get the tiniest bit sciencey here but listen up because it's important: you've got monosaccharides, oligosaccharides and polysaccharides.

A monosaccharide is the simplest form of sugar (mono meaning 'one', saccharide meaning 'sugar'). Glucose is a monosaccharide. Oligosaccharide is the name for a chain of two to three saccharides (oligo means 'a few'). Table sugar (sucrose) and the main sugar found in milk (lactose) are examples of oligosaccharides. Polysaccharides means 'many sugars' and refers to long and complex chains of sugar molecules. The trendy term for these guys is complex carbohydrates*, and some common food examples include starchy or fibrous vegetables.

The reason for that chemistry lesson was to reiterate my point that not all carbohydrates are equal or evil; they all serve a purpose for differing reasons and functions within the body. Fast-digesting sugars can provide quick energy for the body or brain, whereas complex, fibrous carbs can help to slow down the digestion process, leaving us feeling fuller for longer. Fibre can also help to move toxins and mucus through the gastrointestinal tract (not the sexiest image, but still important).

*I personally dislike the term 'simple' and 'complex' because it leads us erroneously to believe that one is superior to the other. If that were the case, then bread would be technically healthier than fruit, given that fruit is very often termed a simple sugar (due to its fructose content). However, fruit contains some powerful vitamins and minerals that bread just cannot compete with – so in this case it would be silly to opt for complex over simple.

Interestingly, the carbs you consume are eventually converted into glucose (a simple sugar). This is because it's the body's main source of fuel, so much so that it even converts protein (more specifically amino acids) into glucose if it is running low, in a process called glucogenesis. And all this time we thought glucose was the devil. It's really not, but like anything in excess, it can cause issues.

But won't carbs make me fat?
Like all of the macronutrients, carbohydrates in and of themselves don't 'make you fat'. Excessive calorie consumption can make you fat.

In fact, some studies have shown that the body chooses to store excessive dietary fat more efficiently than it does excessive carbohydrates – simply put, eating too much avocado could lead to fat storage more easily than overeating sweet potato.

Which carbohydrates should you consume?
Well the answer is one you've probably been told before – eat as close to nature as possible 95 per cent of the time. Refined foods, although very often delicious, are usually lower in micronutrients and fibre and higher in calories and simple sugars.

Now, does that make refined carbohydrates BAD? No. Vilifying foods is bad because it makes us feel restricted, which I believe is a recipe for yo-yo dieting and eventual binge eating. Labelling anything bad just makes you want it more (like the bad boy in school... just me then?). So rather than stigmatising and slating refined foods I'm simply going to suggest that 95 per cent of your food comes from whole, unrefined food ingredients – not because it's 'cleaner' (another word I'm not a huge

BENEFITS OF CARBOHYDRATE CONSUMPTION

Many carbohydrate-rich foods contain fibre, and I'm sure I'm speaking for everyone here when I say we all feel good when we are 'regular'. However, fibre contributes to much more than just a good poo; adequate intake of fibre can help to lower blood sugar, and in long-term studies has been shown to reduce the risk of colon cancer. Fibre is also associated with a lower risk of obesity. Fibre really is amazing. You can't get it from meat or dairy; it comes from plants.

Carbs increase satiety through a few different mechanisms – soluble fibre being one of them – which help to keep food in your stomach for longer by forming a gel within the gut; think oats and how deliciously gooey they get.

Carbs make us a better person; carbohydrate consumption supports brain function and helps to stimulate feel-good hormones such as serotonin – ever been around someone on a low-/no-carb diet? That stuff breaks up relationships.

fan of) but because it's going to fuel your body more effectively with important micronutrients and fibre that are required for optimal functioning of the body.

That other 5 per cent leeway that I am referring to is for sanity and life enjoyment. It is not to say that you should go out and 'eat all the pizzas'. However, there is a lot of enjoyment to be had from eating, and sometimes that enjoyment comes from a delicious dose of fully refined crème brûlée that is healthy for the soul.

If you were standing in front of me, asking me about my carbohydrate recommendations for YOU, they would greatly depend upon your personal preference (as well as your goals, body type, genetics, lifestyle, activity level, etc.).

As I have mentioned before, what good is the BEST diet if you can't actually sustain it? Choosing the best carbohydrates for your body should always involve acknowledging which ones you actually LIKE the most, as well as the ones that are the most nutrient dense. Broccoli is extremely healthy, but does it excite you as much as bread? Probably not. So we have to find a happy medium.

The table opposite shows my favourite carbohydrate foods – I have divided them into fibrous, starchy and fruity ingredients.

How much to have from each column
The British Dietetic Association suggests that you have five servings of fruit and vegetables per day, with three coming from veg and two coming from fruit. Think of your fruit and vegetables as your multivitamin, with each colour representing a different nutrient. It's important to aim for the rainbow so that you get a huge range of micronutrients.

Wholegrain consumption is a little trickier to define; the British Dietetic Association states that *'There is currently no advice on what amount of wholegrains to eat in the UK but many experts in other countries say to aim for three servings a day'* [10], with each cooked serving being anywhere between 30 and 120g.

Some people feel great consuming more servings of grain per day, whereas others feel bloated and lethargic. This is why it's imperative to listen in to your body and the physical responses you receive from your food – despite what the media or even the

CARBOHYDRATE NIRVANA

FIBROUS/NON-STARCHY VEGETABLES	STARCHY VEGETABLES, GRAINS AND LEGUMES	FRUIT
These contain a small amount of starch, are low in calories, have loads of fibre and are PACKED with vitamins and minerals to keep your body functioning like the superhero that you really are.	These are higher in carbohydrate content and provide the body with glycogen to support muscle growth.	While it contains fructose (which in high amounts – more than 50g – can be dangerous to the body) fruit contains important vitamins and minerals that far outweigh the fructose. Whole fruits are also fibrous, which is why it's best to eat fruit whole, rather than in juices where you lose the fibre and just drink the fructose.
Beetroots and chard Brassicas (broccoli, Brussels sprouts, cabbage, cauliflower, kale) Carrots Courgette (zucchini) and other summer squashes Garlic Green beans Leafy greens (spinach, rocket, dandelion greens, pak choi, watercress, etc.) Mangetout Peppers (capsicums)	All potatoes, including sweet potatoes, white potatoes, taro, cassava Grains: oats, rye, couscous, barley, wild rice Legumes, including mung beans, kidney beans, adzuki beans, peanuts, peas (yes that's right, peas are high in protein and carbs, but low in fat) and lentils Pumpkin and winter squashes (they're in this category but are actually relatively low in carbohydrates) Quinoa Rice (I personally enjoy both white and brown)	All fruit!

experts say. Interestingly, when it comes to fat loss, some studies [11] have shown that there is no significant difference between low-fat vs. low-carb diets and the most important thing in regards to fat loss still appears to be a calorific deficit (eating under your daily energy expenditure).

Carbohydrates in the form of vegetables contain an array of vitamins and minerals (as well as macronutrients) that are vital to optimal functioning of the body. The best advice I can provide is to ensure that you are consuming a range of different grains and vegetables in your servings. You will notice in the 28-day reset plan that we consume various types across the recipes to ensure the intake of those important micronutrients.

Fat

Like carbs, fat at one stage was also wrongly accused of making us fat and even killing us prematurely, and, because of that, low-fat diets hit the scene like Billie Jean. We threw away the egg yolk, swapped butter for margarine and filled our new low-fat foods with excess sodium and sugar to make up for the lack of taste.

While fat takes a little more energy to burn than carbohydrates and protein (1g fat is equal to 9 calories whereas 1g protein or carbohydrate equals 4 calories), it is still vital to the functioning of our system. Funnily enough, eating the right amount and type of fat can actually help to reduce body fat. 'Good' fats are very closely linked to supporting hormone regulation, which we know governs metabolism. In addition to metabolism, balanced hormone production will also support other systems within the body, including the reproductive system.

As with certain amino acids, there are fatty acids, found in 'healthy' fats, which are essential to the body (meaning the body can't produce its own). The essential fatty acids help to produce omega-3s and omega-6s, which play a huge role in various functions within the body. Omega-3s, particularly those found in marine animals in the form of EPA and DHA, support brain function and fat metabolisation, as well as reduce inflammation, which has been shown to improve various autoimmune diseases. Omega-6s are important for skin and hair growth, and support bone health, regulate metabolism and maintain reproductive health. Meat, chicken, eggs, nuts, wheat, most vegetable oils – and so many more ingredients – contain omega-6s, so they are very common.

Western diets lean towards excessive omega-6 consumption, and this has been shown to actually increase the risk of chronic inflammatory diseases. The ideal ratio of omega-3 to omega-6 is 1:1 – don't worry if you're feeling a little overwhelmed, I was too when I heard this. This is why omega-3 supplementation, particularly if you're not consuming fish, might be a good idea; more on that on page 73.

It's vital to obtain your dietary fat from 'healthy' fats, comprising mostly mono- and polyunsaturated fats (olive oil, avocados, macadamias, fatty fish) and some saturated fats (butter, ghee, animal fats and yummy coconut oil). The British Nutrition Foundation recommends no more than 70g fat per day for women and 90g for men, with no more than 30–50g of that coming from saturated fats.

The most important thing to remember when it comes to healthy fat consumption is avoiding trans fats (as much as sanely possible). Trans fats are oils that have undergone the hydrogenation process to stop them from going rancid and to increase the shelf life of the product they are used in. Yet they are extremely toxic to the body and should be avoided. Abstain from products like margarine and highly processed junk foods.

Unfortunately, there are no legal requirements for companies to label trans fats on packaging. However, they do have to label all ingredients, so check the packaging for the word 'hydrogenated' or even 'partially hydrogenated'.

Overleaf is a table outlining some of my favourite fats and their benefits. Of course, there are many different fats out there that you can and should integrate into your diet; these are just some of my personal loves – they are easy to integrate into a lunchbox or to cook with at dinner.

FAT IS THE NEW BLACK

Especially saturated fat. In the past, saturated fat was blamed for wreaking havoc on our bodies, but new research is suggesting that there is little to no correlation between saturated fat and heart disease. In fact, it seems that saturated fat is actually healthy and important for the body. Of course, like anything, it's key to get the balance right; overeating uber-healthy coconut oil could still cause fat gain.

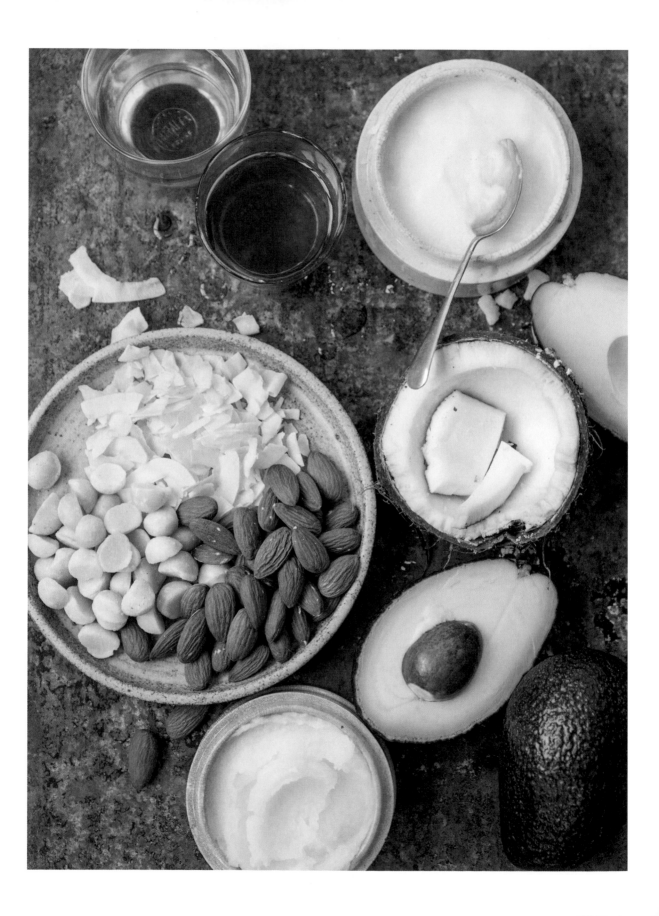

NUTRITIOUS AND DELICIOUS FATS

FOOD	TYPE	BENEFITS
Avocado	Unsaturated	Avocados are a great source of vitamin K, as well as folate, and contain more potassium than a banana. Be careful not to overdo it though: a 200g avocado contains 29g fat. As trendy as avocados are, chomping down on three a day is not a balanced approach.
Macadamia nuts	Unsaturated	I might be a little biased on these guys because they come from my home, Australia. Macadamias were once criticised for their high fat content in comparison to other nuts, however they actually contain the lowest amount of omega-6s out of all the nuts. Remember omega-6 in excess can cause inflammation and increase the risk of certain chronic inflammatory diseases, so if you love your nuts, macadamias might be a better option. They also contain high amounts of vitamin B1 as well as magnesium.
Almonds	Unsaturated	Almonds seem to be the most popular nuts ever. They are lower in fat than macadamias, and high in magnesium, calcium and iron. Almonds are quite moreish so be careful not to overeat them. 100g almonds contain 49g fat.
Oily fish	Unsaturated	While the sustainability of the fishing industry can be something of a moral dilemma, oily fish contain high amounts of omega-3s which, as mentioned, play a huge part in brain function and metabolism. They also contain anti-inflammatory properties, and some, such as mackerel, herring and sardines, are considered sustainable species when fished responsibly. Oily fish also include salmon. It is possible to supplement omega-3, however it's really important to be scrupulous when choosing the brand. As a polyunsaturated fat it can go rancid quite quickly if overprocessed. Always research the brand and its methodology. NOTE: You can also get vegan omega-3s that are made from the algae that fish eat.

FOOD	TYPE	BENEFITS
Flaxseed oil	Unsaturated	An amazing oil that is high in magnesium, manganese and even vitamin B1, 3 tablespoons flaxseed oil contain 6338mg omega-3s. However, as with all oils that are liquid at room temperature, if overheated it can become rancid, and flaxseed oil seems to be highly susceptible to rancidity. Check that it does not taste bitter; it should be clean and nutty tasting. Flaxseed oil has shown dual effectiveness in both constipation and diarrhoea – great! It's best used in smoothies.
Coconut flesh	Saturated	I'm obsessed with coconuts, but then I am an islander and my mum practically raised me on them. Apart from the benefits of medium chain triglycerides which you'll read more about below in coconut oil, coconut flesh is high in fibre, as well as potassium and manganese. It can also provide 13 per cent of your RDI of iron. Coconuts and avocados have seen a huge growth in popularity recently (which is great because they are full of nutrients), however their nutrient content does not negate their fat content, so it's important to be mindful of over-consumption. The same rules to fat intake apply.
Coconut oil	Saturated	The research coming out about coconut oil and its positive effect on our body is quite profound. Coconut oil is high in medium chain fatty acids, which are easily broken down and used as energy by the body. These fatty acids are converted into ketones, which are showing to have positive effects on epilepsy and Alzheimer's.
Butter	Saturated	Butter is high in butyric acid, which has shown to benefit metabolism and reduce inflammation. There are some small studies now to show butyric acids support IBS as well. I love to cook with butter because of its delicious taste. However, it is dense in calories, so don't overdo it.
Extra virgin olive oil (cold pressed)	Saturated	Cold pressed extra virgin olive oil is extremely good for you, mostly because of its phenolic compound content, in particular oleocanthal which is found in high amounts. It possesses similar anti-inflammatory properties to ibuprofen[12].

Balancing macronutrients

Now that you know a little more about macronutrients and their various roles within the body, the next logical step is to look at how much of each macronutrient we need to consume. Unfortunately, you would be hard pressed to find a more debated topic, because balancing macronutrients really differs with each body and is goal-dependent, so it's difficult to suggest what will exactly work for you.

A very active young athlete will require more carbohydrates then an office worker who spends 80 per cent of their day in a chair, training no more than twice per week. Genetics can also play a part: some people just feel and function better with a higher carbohydrate diet, while others can't get enough of that buttery, fatty goodness and can feel sluggish after carbohydrates.

This is why listening to your own body is key – how do you feel after eating the various macronutrients?

The one thing that most agree on is the need to maintain protein levels – because remember, we can store carbohydrates and fats, but our body has no way to store protein or amino acids; it requires a constant supply.

High-protein diets have been shown to help maintain muscle mass during calorie deficit diets. If you're trying to lose body fat, it's important to maintain your protein levels so that you preserve the muscle you already have and just lose the fat.

In my experience, most people don't eat enough protein, nor do they consume enough greens. So the Vertue Method is based around helping you hit both protein and vegetable requirements first.

So, how much protein do you need?

The Reference Nutrient Intake (RNI), set by the British Nutrition Foundation, states that adults need to consume 0.75g protein per kilogram of body weight each day.

However, there are also studies to suggest that 1.3–1.6g protein per kilogram of body weight is required to stimulate maximal protein synthesis, as well as conclusive studies to suggest that protein intake over 1.8g per kilogram of body weight ceases to yield any further protein synthesis.

Unfortunately, there is no definitive answer. You really have to follow a little of what the research recommends as well as a little of what your own intuition tells you. The formula that I use for the Vertue Method is generally on the higher side of protein intake recommendations, for a few reasons. The first is because most people I know struggle to get enough so I want to accommodate for a little human error. Overeating protein (provided it's within your calorific demands) will not lead to fat gain as easily as overeating carbohydrates and fats.

Secondly, you'll be doing resistance-based training four times a week, as well as HIIT cardio twice a week. The guidelines that are suggested by the British Nutrition

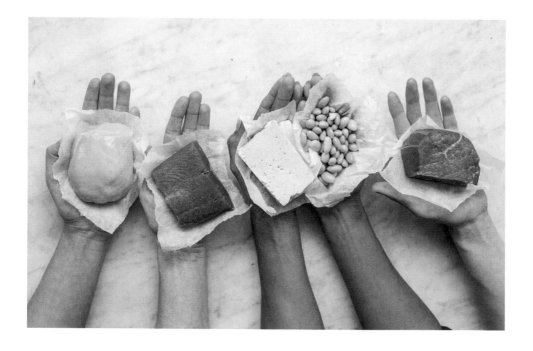

Nourish

Foundation clearly state that their recommendations are not based on training individuals. A slightly higher protein intake can support fat loss and encourage muscle development (remember, for sculpting and toning, not bulking). It takes into account the fact that you'll be very active, will be undertaking a regular weight training practice and are eating to develop strength.

What about carbs and fats?
The British Dietetic Association suggests that we should consume around 50 per cent of our daily calories from carbohydrates and no more than one third of our calories from fat.

To help facilitate some extra fat loss I will have you consume your carbohydrates around weights workout days when muscle glycogen requires replenishment.

The Vertue Method food plan contains mostly wholefood and minimally processed sources of carbohydrates and fats, to optimise nutrient density of the foods.

Again, I have decided to keep all the sexy mathematical formulas at the back of this book. If you want to get specifically geeky about the macronutrient requirements for your body, you can check those out at the back (see page 262). Instead of having you weigh your food, all you have to do is ensure you're getting enough protein daily. You will do this by making sure you add enough protein to the salads, bowls and green dinners. The shakes and breakfasts all contain 20–25g of protein – so you will fill in the gaps by adding your palm-sized serving of protein to the Vertueous Veggie Box, Booty Bowls and Lean Green dinners. (NOTE: if you are using plant-based, vegan protein sources, you will be adding two palm-sized servings to make up for protein requirements.)

VERTUEOUS HEALTH HACK
Hitting protein targets can be tricky. I keep ziplock bags of my favourite protein powder in my handbag so that if I'm ever low on protein, rather than reaching for a sugary nut bar, I just make a quick shake with some coconut water. It certainly looks dodgy carrying around a bag of white powder but it's worth the strange looks. It always helps me to hit my protein targets.

Micronutrients

The World Health Organization lovingly deems micronutrients as the 'magic wands' that enable the body to produce enzymes, hormones and other substances essential for proper growth and development. They are labelled micronutrients because they are required in much smaller amounts. However, just a small deficiency in any of them can cause severe imbalances and effects within the body, including stunted growth in children and increased risk of various diseases in adulthood.

Micronutrients refer to vitamins (vitamins A, B complex, C, D, E, K), carotenoids, choline and minerals (calcium, chlorine, magnesium, phosphorus, potassium, sodium and sulfur, as well as trace minerals).

Foods that contain a large amount of these micronutrients are often called nutrient dense foods, and although this isn't necessarily a scientific term, I think it helps you to decide what foods will give you the best bang for your buck. Highly processed foods are often low in nutrients as the process of refining the ingredients can greatly diminish the quantity of these delicate vitamins and minerals.

4. ADEQUATE HYDRATION

I don't really need to remind you of this one do I? Hydration is key because our bodies are made up of up to 65 per cent water (a little more in children). Water is required for brain function as well as almost every metabolic function in the body.

If you're still not convinced, I will tell you that adequate hydration can lead to better muscle definition. Why? Because your body will be hydrated enough that it won't 'hold onto' water, which will help you to drop that 'water weight' that's getting in the way of your six-pack shining through.

Hydration is hugely dependent upon your environment, your activity levels and also, of course, your body. If you're a profuse sweater, then obviously you're going to need a little more water. Common sense is key. The British Dietetic Association suggests 1.6 litres for women and 2 litres for men per day. Cups of tea and coffee do count, as do some foods that are higher in water content, like watermelon and cucumber. However, I personally believe in the powers of pure water. Other types of drink will contain ingredients such as caffeine and sugar which aren't great for you in high amounts.

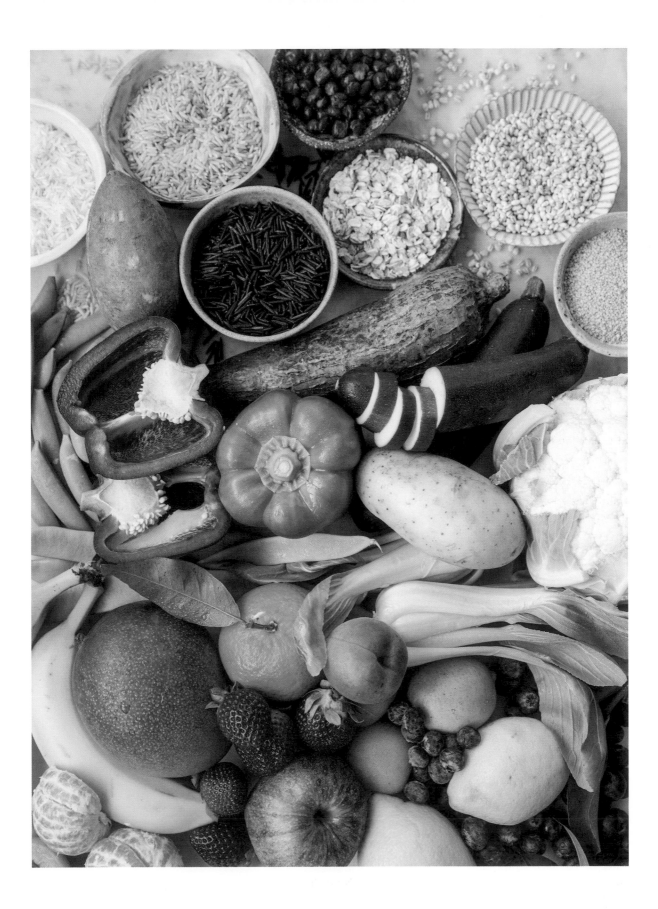

For the Vertue Method plan I would really like you to be consuming a minimum of 2 litres a day as you will be doing rigorous lifting.

One way to check whether your hydration is to look at the colour of your urine: it should be either clear or very lightly yellow. If it is as foamy as the sea and as dark as a pint of lager, chances are you need to drink more.

5. INTUITION

Intuition tends to have an air of dogma attached to it and can sound a little esoteric. However, I assure you I mean it in a practical sense. Intuition is the ability to understand something instinctively, without the need for conscious reasoning. However, in the case of diet, I am referring to you paying greater attention to the symptoms and messages from your body. Learning to listen in and understand whether you require food, water or just a little movement, is going to play a huge part in sustaining a healthy life and body.

There are currently 7.4 billion different bodies on the planet. Different circumstances, lifestyles and genetics play a role in how we each process food, and if you rely purely on the current accepted science you cut yourself off from the most important information – that provided to you by your incredibly intelligent body.

In order to stay healthy you must stay up to date with two things: firstly, what contemporary science says about the food you should consume and, just as importantly, what your body says to you about the food you consume.

After every meal, observe and listen to the various messages you receive from your body. The 28-day reset plan is designed to help you pick up on those messages better.

A very common problem within the fitness industry is that many people suggest it's their way or no way. Very often someone has experienced the benefits of eliminating gluten or going 'low-carb', and suddenly everyone should do it. However, that's just not the case; we are all different and we need to take that into account. Do the research but, ultimately, you are going to have to make the decision about what feels right and most effective in your body.

In this day and age of information overload and trusting technology over our own intelligent bodies and minds, we have lost connection to our intuition. This is why I have made intuition itself one of the main aspects of achieving a healthy body.

Quinoa is a very trendy grain to consume right now; it's high in protein and is gluten-free. However, if you feel bloated and uncomfortable after consuming it, then it's probably not the food for you. Some people can tolerate dairy really well, whileothers clear the room with their flatulence after a single drop of milk to the tongue.

After every meal, observe and listen to the various messages you receive from your body. The 28-day reset plan is designed to clear the proverbial slate as a means to help you pick up on those messages a little better. Giving up alcohol and then reintroducing it back into your life is a really interesting way to notice the true effects of it.

The bottom line is that I don't want you to just take my word for it. Try it all, but be observant and trust your gut (literally).

VERTUEOUS HEALTH HACK

I know it can be hard to drink water, particularly if you live in a cold climate, but the body actually requires adequate hydration to keep you warm as well. My health hack for consuming enough water is to have a huge 2-litre jug on your desk. Make it a goal to finish the jug before you leave work that afternoon. For those of you working on the run, grab one of those BRITA bottles that you can refill – that way you have filtered water on the go: no excuses.

RULES ABOUT THE C-WORD: CAFFEINE!

Those of you who follow me on social media will know that I am an avid lover of coffee and I defiantly promote its benefits. Both tea and coffee are high in antioxidants and caffeine has been shown to support a range of health benefits, including the following:

- Benefits to cognition and memory consolidation [13]
- Positive effects on Alzheimer's disease [14] [15]
- Boosting energy levels and reducing time until exhaustion during aerobic exercise [16]
- A natural stimulant that reduces tiredness and improves concentration
- Causing an increase in dopamine, the neurotransmitter associated with motor control, motivation and desire

NO WONDER WE LOVE COFFEE…

However, in saying all that, in excess (500mg and above), caffeine can cause insomnia, adrenal fatigue, dehydration, tremors, anxiety, addiction, increased blood pressure and stomach ulcers. So even though I love to promote the benefits of coffee, I am well aware of its potential side effects if it's abused.

I am not going to take coffee or tea away from you, I only ask that you make a few minor changes to the way in which you use it:

1. No caffeine after 2pm – Some of us are more sensitive to caffeine than we realise, and reducing our caffeine intake in the afternoon will help us chill out before bed. Sleep is key for recovery and cognitive function, and while you're on this plan (and hopefully for the rest of your life) you'll want to sleep soundly and deeply. Another reason to limit caffeine intake in the afternoon is to train yourself to reach for water or herbal tea when you feel that 3pm slump instead of a cookie and cappuccino.

2. Keep it simple and pure – I used to only drink mochas (chocolate and coffee: is there any better match?). However, I may as well have just asked for some coffee with my sugar. Drink black coffee with some milk (if needed) rather than an orange mocha frappuccino, which will be laced with all kinds of highly refined sugars.

3. No more than two cups of coffee (or three cups of tea) per day – It is recommended you avoid having more than 200mg caffeine per day. It's difficult to know exactly how much caffeine goes into each cup of coffee, as various brewing and harvesting techniques can change the caffeine content, but roughly one cup of filtered coffee contains 140mg caffeine and one cup of tea approximately 75mg. What is also important to remember is that addiction and reliance on coffee can occur with as little as 100mg per day. So, try not to abuse this socially acceptable psychoactive drug. Use it sparingly and wisely.

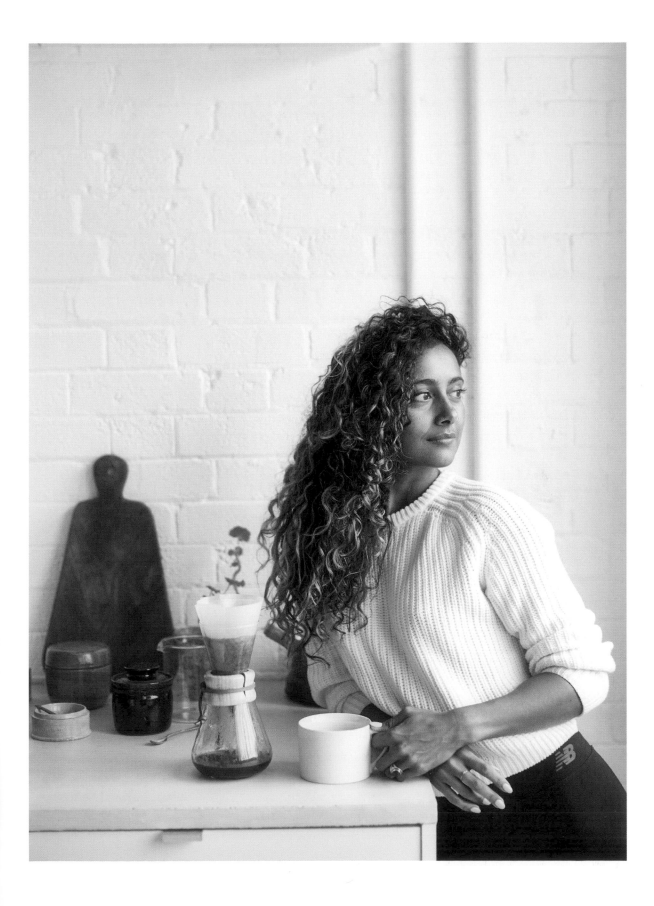

PART TWO: MEDITATION

Meditation has saved my sanity. As an overthinking people-pleaser my mind was both relentless and assiduous. In Sydney, all the time I spent in nature gave me the space between thoughts so that I never felt overwhelmed by them. So, as you can imagine, moving from a lifestyle that included daily surf sessions and lunch breaks in national parks, to a big and busy city like London, was a huge cultural and environmental shock for me. It actually affected me much more than I had originally and naively thought it would. In fact, if I had known just how much I would miss the ocean, I might never have moved in the first place, but I now thank my lucky stars that I did, because it was that unruffling of my feathers that actually helped me understand the true value of daily meditation.

WHAT IS IT?

Meditation is a very general term for fairly different practices. Asking what is meditation is similar to asking what training is; it really depends on the type. However, ultimately the goal of meditation is to connect you so deeply to the present moment that you are no longer lost in the relentless and incessant movement of the mind. By focusing all your awareness on a single activity or point of focus you can ultimately quieten the noise of those persistent thoughts, creating 'space' to process potentially overwhelming thoughts and emotions.

Meditation is not limited to just simply sitting still. It can be experienced while playing an instrument, moving through a yoga sequence or performing a healing movement like t'ai chi.

The prerequisite of meditation, however, is that the movement or activity is not detrimental to yourself or others. You can experience meditational-like states while playing football or sprinting; however, those kinds of activities are obviously quite depleting on the physical system.

Meditation has the power to quite literally transform your mind. That may sound a little vague and abstruse, but scientific studies have shown that a regular meditation practice can change the physiology of the brain by changing patterns within the brain, ultimately modifying various neurological pathways.

A consistent meditation practice has been shown to reduce activity in the 'me' centre of the brain as well as its connection to bodily sensation and the fear centres

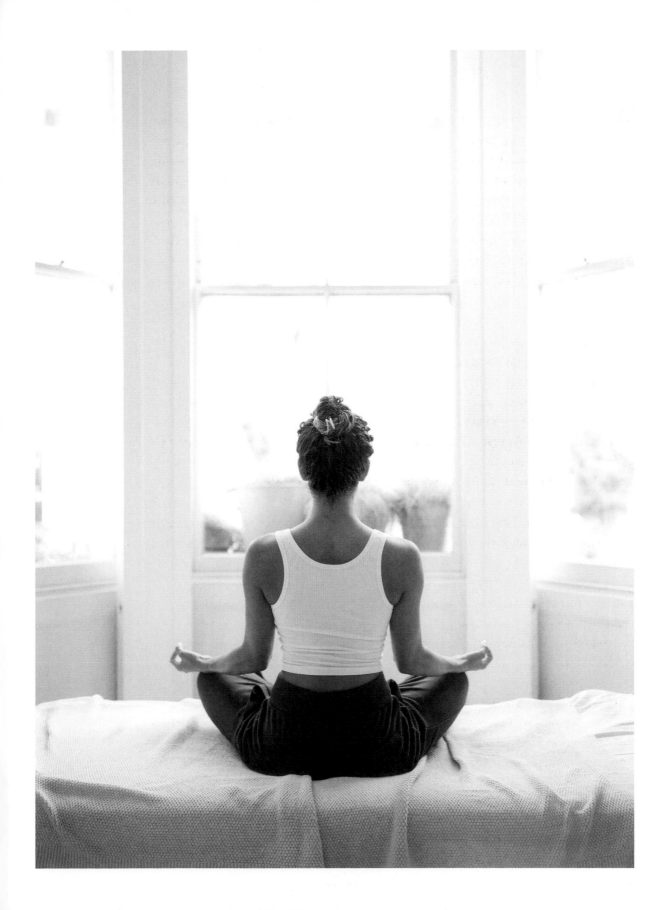

of the brain – this is one of the reasons that experts believe meditation can help to reduce anxiety. Meditation also helps to cultivate a more mindful approach to your life. Mindfulness is essentially increased awareness.

WHAT MEDITATION ISN'T

Always relaxing – I realise this looks like a massive contradiction. A lot of people confuse the outcome of meditation with the actual practice of meditation. Sitting in a cross-legged position for a designated period of time while trying to stop thought by focusing on the breath is for some people relaxing. However, for others, being made to sit still for 15 minutes with nothing but relentless internal chatter and a nose whistle is just downright torture.

So meditation over time, if practised regularly, can help you to relax through experiencing less daily anxiety. However, the practice itself for many can actually be quite confronting and uncomfortable. It's really worth knowing that, because if you judge the benefits of meditation on its immediate effect, you will most likely give up in the first 60–180 seconds. Sound familiar? Give it another go.

A quick fix – In the same way that one day of clean eating won't make you leaner, one meditation session won't make you a zen master; it won't even help you be as calm as Kanye. In order for meditation to take full effect it must be practised regularly – I'm talking on a daily basis here. 10 minutes a day is going to be far more effective than an hour once a month. It takes 24 days to change a habit; the Vertue Method asks that you practise every day for 28 days in the hope that it will transform your mental patterns beyond the plan.

A chore –Just like exercise, meditation practice shouldn't feel like a chore. I want you to find reasons to get excited about it. This is why I have offered you three different types of meditation here in this book. Find the one that makes you feel happy and excited to do. If my three fail to uplift you in some way then use a guided meditation from YouTube (some of my favourites are by Thich Nhat Hanh and Abraham Hicks, but you should, of course, find a voice and message that resonates with you) and allow yourself to find joy in the practice. The more you love it, the more you'll do it.

HOW CAN YOU BEGIN TO MEDITATE?

The techniques that I prescribe within this book are geared to those of you who are new to meditation, or who have tried it and hated it.

From my own experience, guided meditations seem to be the best way to develop an initial practice; following on from there it becomes enough simply to listen to calming music and, after that, the breath alone is enough to take you into that deeply calm state.

I am not a meditation guru; the techniques I want to share with you are simply the methods that I have used to help me. If you feel as though you're struggling with the methods I provide, don't give up. Continue your search for the perfect teacher and method. The Vertue Method contains three different types of meditational exercises, outlined on the pages that follow.

Please note you'll need a recording device (I use the Voice Memos app on my phone).

SCIENCE SAYS

This is my favourite part. Because now I get to take a daily hippie-endorsed esoteric practice, and show you some of the incredible research that is proving its validity in modern day society. Sceptics, listen up:

Meditation reduces the symptoms of depression (such as anxiety, rumination, dysfunctional attitudes).[17]

It increases grey matter in the right side of the hippocampus and orbito frontal cortex of meditators, suggesting better processing of emotions and cognitive decision-making.[18]

It also leads to better immune function.[19]

SUN SALUTATION MEDITATION

This is a moving meditation, commonly known in yoga as the Sun Salutation. Record the below script onto your phone, explaining the details very slowly so that your movement matches the pace of a slow breath. Make sure you read everything within this script, including the breath.

The practice

Roll out your mat and come to stand in Tadasana (image 1). Take 5 deep breaths here with your eyes closed to enable your mind to focus. Press play on your recording device to begin.

Inhale – *Reach your arms above your head (2).*

Exhale – *Fold forwards, bringing your hands towards the floor (3).*

Inhale – *Place the hands on the shins, flatten the back and look forwards (4).*

Hold the breath – *Step into a lunge position (5).*

Exhale – *Step into a push-up position* and lower (6).*

Inhale – *Push into the arms to lift your chest and come into a back bend. Keep your knees, hips and thighs off the floor (7).*

Exhale – *Press back into downward facing dog (8). Stay here for 5 breaths. (Breathe on your recording so you can keep the timing of 5 breaths.)*

Inhale – *Bend your knees and look forwards.*

Exhale – *Step the feet to the hands and fold your head towards your shins (9).*

Inhale – *Lift the body and reach up to the sky (10).*

Exhale – *Bring your hands to prayer at the heart (11).*

Repeat the sequence five times.

Who's it for?

• Those who are feeling stiff and tight or sluggish.

• Anyone feeling busy in the mind and requires physical movement to focus upon.

• Great for those who feel restless when meditating.

*Don't worry if you don't have the strength for a full push-up; drop your knees to the floor before lowering your chest.

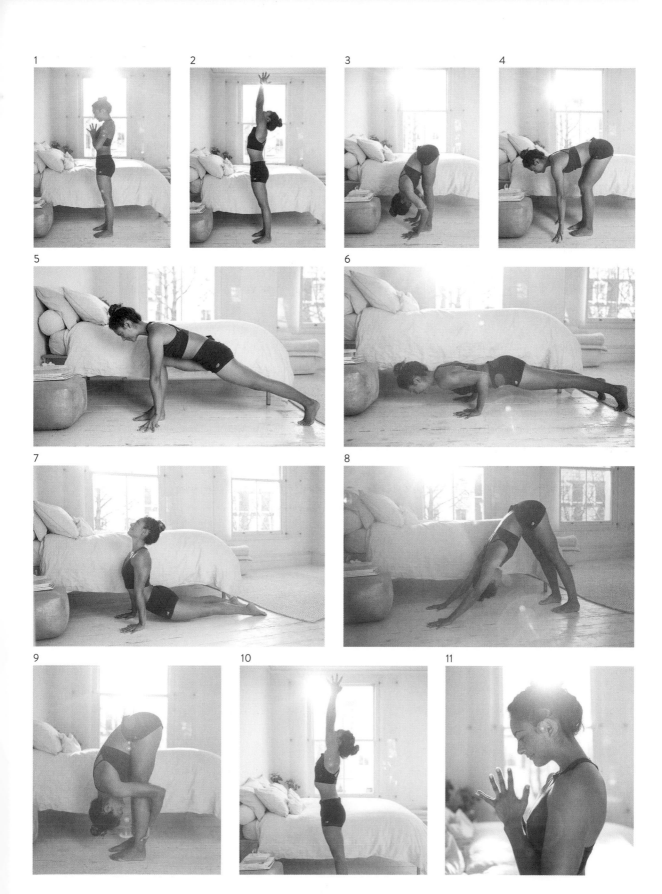

POSITIVE MANTRA MEDITATION

Positive affirmation meditation is one of those practices with which you are either going to really resonate or feel absolutely ridiculous doing. I find this meditation to have been the most powerful practice in my life. It can be likened to positive thinking and pre-visualisation – a technique that when employed and tested on athletes has yielded successful results. As hippie as the concept may seem, visualising a positive outcome has been shown by science to improve results.

The purpose of this meditation is to get your mind and body excited for all the wonderful things to come in the near future. The body doesn't know the difference between your reality and your imagination, which is why your thoughts are so important. If you wake up every morning and reflect on all the things you hate about your body or life, you are starting on the wrong foot. It's difficult to have a good day when you've begun on a negative pretence.

The practice

This meditation is bespoke: you're going to write (and record) a script that you will personalise with the things you want. The script contains breath instruction and is set in the future, anticipating the success that awaits you just around the corner. If you want to quit your job and start your own business, for example, you're going to write a script as though you've already achieved it. You're also going to discuss the things you love about your current life. Keep the script the same for the full 28 days.

The breath instruction is designed to give you space to absorb the positive sentence that you have just heard, as well as the time to refocus the mind and relax the body.

As soon as your morning alarm goes off, sit up in your bed (maybe put your headphones in if someone is lying next to you), place a pillow under your hips and press play on your recording. Close your eyes.

I can't give you a script other than the example opposite. This exercise is extremely personal and, as I mentioned, it's really not for everyone. Personally, I love to imagine and dream up sensational possibilities in my future because it gets me in such a wonderful mood. I also used to practise these sorts of visualisation exercises as a gymnast and dancer before a performance. The pre-visualisation helps to focus the mind and prepare the body towards the successful outcome of a goal. For me, it has always worked. However, if it makes you feel stupid listening to the sound of your own voice, talking about how good your life and body are, I can understand that. Try one of the other two meditation techniques instead.

Here is an example script:

Good morning Sarah,
Let's breathe.

Inhale, exhale.
Inhale, exhale.
Inhale, exhale.

Maintain this deep, slow and rhythmic breath.
Every morning I feel eager to wake up and get into my day.

Inhale, exhale.

I love my flexible and strong body.
It feels so good to [insert your goal].

Inhale, exhale.

My business is successful, so I have the
 chance to fit training in every day.
I feel energised at the thought of processing
 all the challenges that come my way, while
 running my business.

Inhale, exhale.

I love my family. They are so proud of my
 achievements.

Who's it for?
- Anybody who loves to use their imagination.
- Anyone wanting to start their day on a positive note.
- I personally think this one is great for those of you who don't really like traditional meditation. It's really more like a visualisation with some concentration on the breath to keep the nervous system calm and the body relaxed.

BREATH MEDITATION

The breath and the nervous system have a very close relationship – one affects the other. If you are feeling stressed, the rate of your breathing will increase unconsciously, further stimulating the nervous system and leading to potential increases in stress hormones. This would be appropriate if we were running away from something dangerous. However, if the stress is simply coming from a work deadline or a financial debt, we don't need to prepare the body to run, we actually need to stay calm, relaxed and focused. Enter breath meditation. By paying close attention to your breath, while also slowing it down, you not only enter a more meditative state, you stimulate the parasympathetic nervous system (the one that is in charge of sleep, rest, digestion, etc.). Record the below script onto your phone, reading everything, including the breaths, and paying attention to the pauses.

The practice

As soon as your morning alarm goes off, sit up in bed with a straight back, place a pillow under your hips and rest the backs of your hands on your knees. Press play on your recording. Relax your shoulders. Close your eyes.

Inhale, exhale.
Notice the sensations of the breath.
Inhale, exhale.
Feel the expansiveness of the inhale and the relaxation of the exhale.
Inhale, feel full.
Exhale, feel relaxed.

Bring your awareness to the palms of your hands. (*pause to feel the sensation*)
Inhale and imagine breathing in through the palms of your hands. (*pause*)
Exhale and feel the air release through the palms of your hands. (*pause*)
Inhale through the palms of your hands.
Exhale through the palms of your hands.
   (*pause to feel the sensation*)
Inhale.
Exhale.
Now bring your awareness to your ribcage.
Inhale, feel the ribs expand. Shift the awareness to your shoulders.
Exhale, feel the shoulders relax.
Inhale, ribs expand.
Exhale, shoulders relax.
Inhale, ribs expand.
Exhale, shoulders relax. (*pause*)
Next we will count the inhale and exhale.
   You're going to **inhale** for 3 seconds.
   And **exhale** for 6 seconds.
Inhale for one, two, three.
Exhale for six, five, four, three, two, one.
Inhale for one, two, three.
Exhale for six, five, four, three, two, one.
Continue this process without my guidance for another five rounds, counting them yourself. (*Pause to allow for these breaths; when you make the recording, do this breathing so that the timing for the pause is correct*)
Allow yourself to remain here for a few moments, noticing the sensations in your body. Remember, every morning we are born again; it's what we do today that matters most. Gently open your eyes. Have a wonderful day.

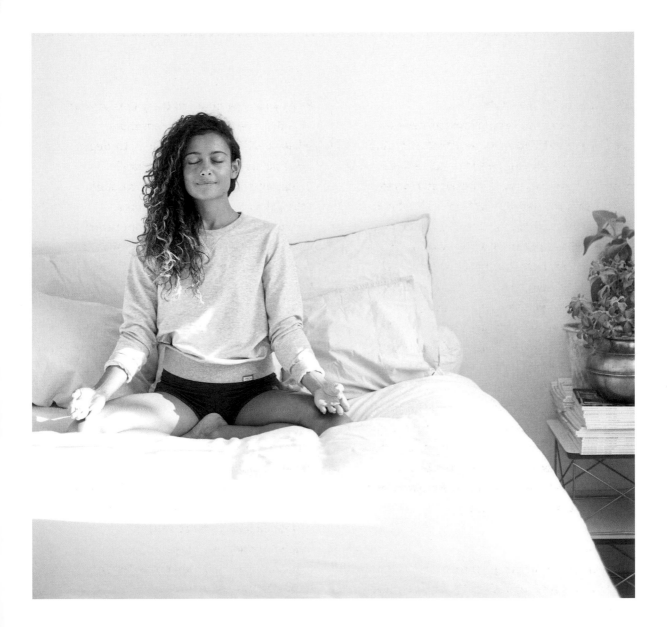

Who's it for?

• Everyone. Paying attention to the breath and practising how to slow it down is an ancient practice used among various schools of meditation and yoga.

• Busy minds: the breath becomes a mental landmark for the present moment preventing you from checking off your to-do list).

• When anxiety gets in the driver's seat of your body and mind, this technique can get it out! Those who have suffered from anxiety will know what I mean by that. If you feel anxious, a steady breath focus can work almost immediately. It might not fix the problem, but it can provide temporary relief to regain control and focus.

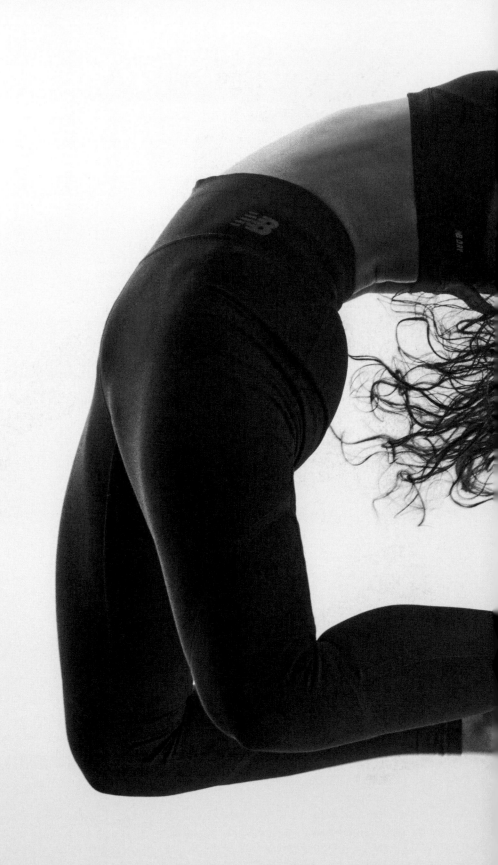

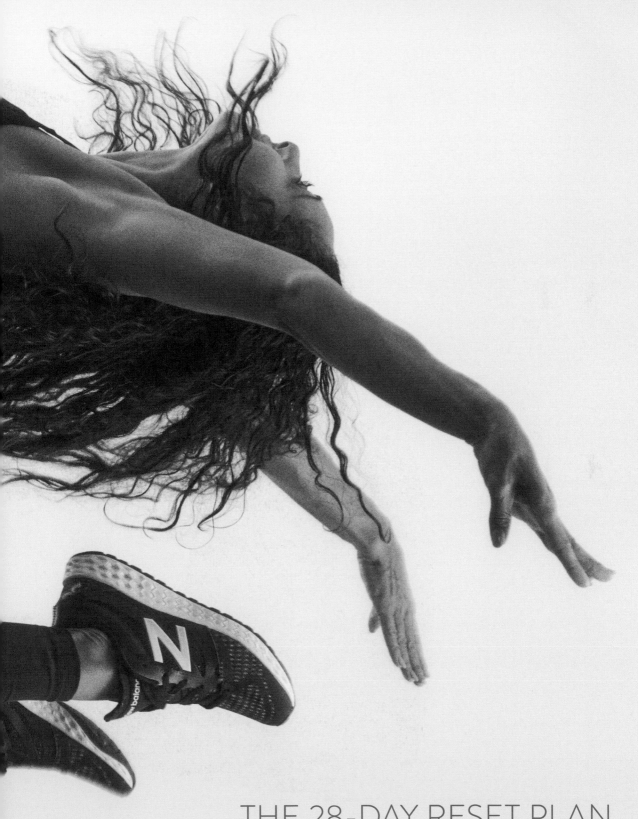

THE 28-DAY RESET PLAN

THE 28-DAY RESET PLAN

You've made it! (Or perhaps you skipped the preceding chapters… I get it, I used to do that too.) Either way, here we are, ready to embark on a transformation. I want to remind you that long-term transformations are physiological adaptations – so building shape (i.e. muscle) and developing and maintaining flexibility both take time; anywhere from three to six months. This programme is designed to reset your mind and establish new healthy habits. Don't get me wrong – you WILL become leaner because, believe it or not, that's the easy part (if you keep to the plan, of course).

This **28-day reset plan** will facilitate the changes that you want IF you stick to the three Cs: **courage, compliancy and consistency.**

Courage: This is always required when we embark on any new way of life, particularly one of this nature. You may feel silly doing some of these things, as we all have at some stage in our lives when trying to learn a new skill. The key is to approach it with a childlike heart, full of ambition but with a heavy dose of playfulness.

Compliancy: Should you only do half the things I ask of you, then you should expect half the results. If you really want to achieve this, 100 per cent compliancy is necessary.

Consistency: Buddha says a jug fills drop by drop. Consistency is about achieving small goals on a daily basis, rather than giant goals once every three months. Smaller goals are less overwhelming and might feel less impressive in the short term, but achieving these small goals consistently is what will amount to true transformation.

HOUSEKEEPING RULES

When I say 'house' I'm referring to your body, and I just have a few rules that I need you to abide by in order to manifest benefits. No matter how much we say that we want to be told what to do when it comes to diet and exercise, the inner child in us rebels and refuses to play along – it is human nature! For that reason I want to explain the rules and why they will benefit you. They will help you to stay motivated.

1. Set your intentions – Before you go out and buy your courgettes and kettlebells, I want you to reflect upon your intentions for this 28-day reset and why you want to embark on it. This isn't going to be a small 'sit-and-think'; I would like you to use a notebook as a training diary and write the different short- and long-term goals you have for embarking on this journey with me. Start with small short-term goals, and

then take a moment to write down some of the more substantial improvements that you would like to feel (and see). Your smaller goal might be making sure you bring your salad to work every day or waking up early enough to make time for training. Your bigger intentions are those soul-satisfying things – like becoming strong enough to perform full push-ups or comfortably touch your toes, or it could be developing the energy to run around with your children, or to feel calmer in your life or to simply fit into your favourite pair of jeans. The bigger picture helps us to remain motivated for life. When you hit the middle or even the end of the 28 days, reviewing this larger intention may just be the key to keeping your head and heart 'in the game'. Review these intentions frequently. I know that it may seem like a redundant and potentially time-wasting exercise, when you already know that you are eager to begin, but I guarantee that this will be a source for unwavering motivation as your 28 days come to a close.

2. No alcohol – This is not because I don't want you to have fun. It's actually because I do want you to have fun! From a physical perspective alcohol is going to inhibit your fat loss – there's just no getting around that. Take a full break from it for 28 days and I promise the benefits alone will bring you mental and physical clarity that will motivate you to steer clear of it. *(See alcohol metabolisation in the Glossary on page 263 for more motivation.)*

3. Daily meditation – This is non-negotiable: I don't care if you have to do it on a London tube with your head buried in somebody's armpit: close your eyes and get mindful. I have provided three meditation techniques (see pages 88–93), so choose whichever best suits your situation. In the same way that skipping your workout will hinder your physical results, skipping meditation will limit your mental results.

4. Pantry and fridge clean-out – Before you embark on this journey it will be best to have a clean-out of processed and refined food you have in the house. Please don't throw it away; perhaps donate it to a neighbour or look for a food donation box. This includes the brown and red sauces that you might be in the habit of pouring all over your meals. This has nothing to do with calories (although it will make a difference to them), it's actually because I want your taste buds to reset to appreciate unprocessed foods. Processed foods are just quite addictive and not optimal for the body, and the only way to get off them is to cleanse the palate.

HOW TO APPROACH THE PLAN

Tear out this chart, or photocopy it and put it on the fridge so you have a nice clear overview of the next 28 days.

ACTIVITY	MON	TUES	WEDS
MEDITATION	Daily meds	Daily meds	Daily meds
DRINK UP	500ml warm water	500ml warm water	500ml warm water
WORKOUT	VM Workout 1	VM Workout 2	VM Workout 3
BREAKFAST	Breakfast	Breakfast	Breakfast
LUNCH	Vertueous Veggie Box	Vertueous Veggie Box	Vertueous Veggie Box
DINNER	Booty-full Bowl	Booty-full Bowl	Lean Greens
MOBILITY/ FLEXIBILITY	Mobility	Flexibility	Mobility
SMOOTHIE	Smoothie	Smoothie	Smoothie

THURS	FRI	SAT	SUN
Daily meds	Daily meds	Daily meds	Daily meds
500ml warm water	500ml warm water	500ml warm water	500ml warm water
VM Workout 1	VM Workout 2	VM Workout 3	Walk and rest
Breakfast	Breakfast	Breakfast	Breakfast
Vertueous Veggie Box	Vertueous Veggie Box	Vertueous Veggie Box	Vertueous Veggie Box
Booty-full Bowl	Booty-full Bowl	Lean Greens	Booty-full Bowl
Flexibility	Mobility	Flexibility	Flexibility
Smoothie	Smoothie	Smoothie	Smoothie

YOUR DAILY SCHEDULE

Daily meds – Wake and then sit up and meditate. It's really easy to fall into the habit of using your phone or tablet as a means to 'wake you up'. Checking emails, social media and to-do lists might 'feel' like a good way to alert your mind for the day ahead, but it's not. Meditation first thing can help you to bring a touch of mindfulness to your morning routine and ultimately throughout the day. As we know, meditation has some proven benefits for stress reduction, so you'll have the power to handle your day, whatever it may bring. Choose from one of the three meditation options on pages 88–93.

Drink up – Grab a large glass (500ml) and fill half with hot (not boiling) water and half cold. This will help to rehydrate you after your sleep. Remember, hydration helps to keep our bodies lean, our brains functioning and our skin fresh (and so much more).

But first, coffee – I'm not against coffee or caffeine (see page 82), I just prefer to use it prior to a workout so that I make full use of the energy. Good-quality coffee is filled with antioxidants and caffeine can help to boost the metabolism, promoting fat loss. The reason I haven't put it into the schedule is because I don't want you to think it's a 'have-to' kind of practice. If you don't like coffee, don't drink it. If you do want some coffee, for the next 28 days have an Americano/long black blended with your favourite protein powder (coffee snobs, I know that is blasphemous to you). No creamy, orange, double mocha frappuccinos for the next 28 days please.

Get sweaty – I personally prefer to train in the mornings, however it's totally fine to train in the evenings too, or whenever you feel it fits best into your life. If you train in the morning or around lunchtime, feel free to enjoy a black coffee blended with some coconut oil (or MCT oil – see page 263) and half a scoop of protein to give you a boost prior to your workout. Post-workout I would love you to just take a few deep breaths to calm the body and mind before getting on with your day. This relaxation practice will help to kick-start recovery. Remember to also rehydrate with a large glass (preferably 500ml) of water when you've finished training.

Breakfast – Choose one of the breakfast recipes (pages 202–13). They each contain between 20 and 30g protein. I am a firm believer in protein for breakfast, not so much for body composition but for brain function. Carbohydrates can also have a sleep-inducing (carb coma) effect, which is not always conducive to a productive day!

Lunch – Either choose a Vertueous Veggie Box (pages 217–27) or fill a lunchbox using the guidelines in my Make Your Own Salad list (see page 228). Don't forget your portion of protein.

Dinner – You'll either be consuming a Booty-full Bowl (pages 232–45), which contains starchy carbs, or Lean Greens (pages 246–53), which have no starchy carbs. The variations accommodate for the different workout types you will be doing. On the conditioning and off-training days you will be having Lean Greens.

Mobility/Flexibility – Getting flexible before bed has many benefits, but not all raunchy ones. The reason I have put your Lengthen practices here is that they will help to prepare your body for a deeper sleep. By slowing down the breath, you can stimulate the parasympathetic nervous system (the part of the nervous system that is in charge of rest, sleep, recovery and even digestion).

Sweet-ass Smoothies – Those of you with a sweet tooth will have noticed that I haven't put any desserts in the plan. The truth is, often a 'guilt-free' cacao and date ball contains the same amount of sugar as a crème brûlée, and it just turns into glucose within the body. Instead, I'd rather have you choose one of the easily digested smoothie with a yummy serving of fruit to satisfy sweet cravings and give you some micronutrients.

Bed – No phones, tablets or laptops 30 minutes prior to sleep. Read a book or write a diary entry instead.

KEEPING TRACK

Keeping a diary throughout your 28 days is going to be a big part of what keeps you on track and motivated. Not only will it keep your head in the game (so to speak), it will also help you to see where you are improving; not just aesthetically, but also in the gaining of strength and stamina. In addition to this it will help you to learn about which foods work and don't work for your body right now.

Some research has shown that keeping a diary is not only therapeutic, but can also help to improve cognitive abilities elsewhere in our lives – in very untechnical words, it can 'free up space' within the brain. It also becomes an exercise in self-awareness as you go back and reflect on the journey of thoughts and emotions that you experienced over the 28 days.

Tracking workouts

One thing that can occur with tracking is the habit of getting obsessive with numbers or results. I want you to remember that the tracking emphasis is going to be on how you feel emotionally, mentally and physically – not so much on whether you have or haven't lost weight. In saying that, taking some pictures before and after the 28 days is a great way to see some of the changes that will occur.

How to track

Whenever you train it is worthwhile tracking the weight lifted and the repetitions you managed to complete, as well as adding a quick sentence or two on how you felt, for example tired, happy, strong, sexy AF. You can be as detailed or as brief as you want. This is simply to get you into the habit of paying more attention to how you feel. Below is an example of what your notes might look like:

	EXERCISE	REPS	TEMPO	REST	REPS/ SET	WEIGHT	NOTES / FEELINGS
A1	Kettlebell Goblet Box Squat	12–15	2110	10s	12/14/12	10kg	*Legs feeling stronger, couldn't keep up the repetitions at the end of the last set.*

Keeping a food diary

I don't want you to be thinking about food every second of the day, because the truth is that there is much more to life. However, this programme includes a food plan, so I'm sure it will be on your mind more than usual. Let's turn that into a positive.

I want you to scribble into your diary just a note about what you ate and how it made you feel, e.g. bloated, energised, sluggish, well-digested. The reason for this is that it will strengthen your ability to intuitively eat the foods that best suit you. Many of us don't even realise a certain food type is disagreeing with us until we pay more attention to its effect on us. For example, for anyone with a sensitive gut, broccoli can cause bloating and gas. Does that mean that those people should push on through their flatulence because broccoli is a 'health food'? No. They should choose a different green vegetable to work with that doesn't irritate their digestive ability.

How to take pictures
- Choose plain, comfortable underwear or swimwear.
- Photograph at the same time of day, usually in the morning before meals.
- Try to take photos in natural light, rather than indoor lights, as it will give a clearer image.
- Take photos against a plain background.
- Take a front, side and back photo.
- Only take photos at the beginning and end of your 28 days – don't be an obsessive weirdo who takes pictures of themselves every day; it's not necessary and it will cultivate the wrong mentality.

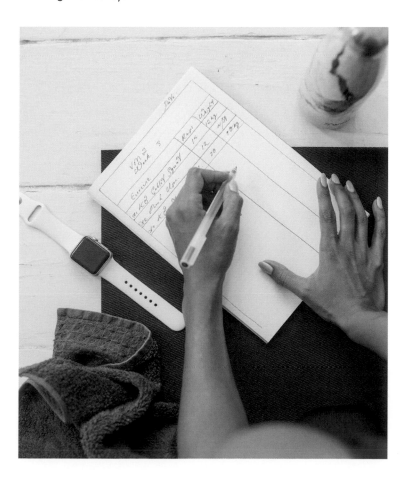

THE MOVEMENT PLAN – THE WORKOUTS

BEFORE YOU TRAIN

Allrighty, here we are. If you skipped over the 'Lift' section, I highly recommend that you flip back to pages 20–31 and review my tips for training and lifting.

In addition to this, I want you to be really sure that you are physically ready and able to undertake a new exercise programme. As a personal trainer and yoga teacher, before embarking on a fitness and health journey with any new client, I will always have them fill out a form called a PARQ. Have a read of the questions below and if you answer 'yes' to even one of them I really urge you to speak to your doctor before getting started.

1. Has your doctor ever said that you have a heart condition and that you should only do physical activity recommended by a doctor?

2. Do you feel pain in your chest when you do physical activity?

3. In the past month, have you had chest pain when you were not doing physical activity?

4. Do you lose your balance because of dizziness or do you ever lose consciousness?

5. Do you have a bone or joint problem (for example, back, knee or hip) that could be made worse by a change in your physical activity?

6. Is your doctor currently prescribing drugs (for example diuretics) for your blood pressure or heart condition?

7. Do you know of any other reason why you should not do physical activity?

If you did answer 'yes', it's not to say that you can't do the exercise, it just flags that you should speak with a physician prior to undertaking something like this. They will be able to look at the programme and tell you what you can or can't do so that you get the most from it, without risking your health.

If you answered 'no' to all of the above, then let's get on with it.

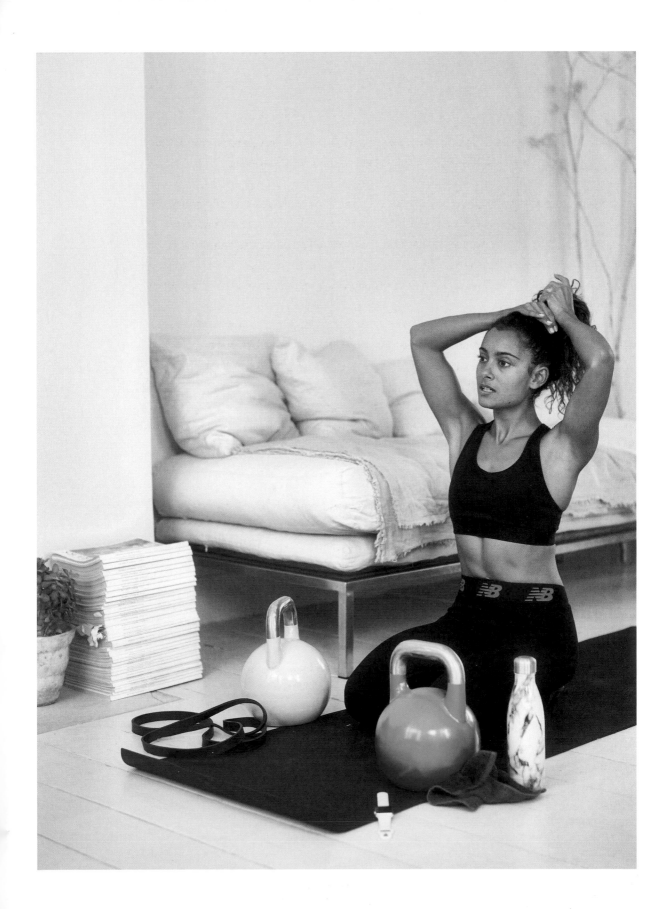

SETTING UP FOR SUCCESS

The moments before a workout are key, because the way in which you prepare is ultimately going to determine how effective the workout is. Follow the tips below to ensure you get the most out of your exercise sessions:

• Have a read of the workout you're about to embark on. You don't have to memorise it, as over the next few weeks you'll obviously get more and more comfortable with the structure, but it's important to know what is coming, how many repetitions, what equipment you'll need, etc.

• Clear up any confusion in advance and clarify before you intensify! If there are any exercises you're not quite sure of when you skim through, have a thorough read of the descriptions and learn the key alignment cues. You don't want to have to stop midway through your workout to learn how to do a reverse crunch. We want to maintain the intensity.

• Lay out all the necessary equipment for the workout, and I'm talking absolutely everything; from kettlebells to music, sweat towels and water. Don't create any excuses to leave the workout zone.

• Get that phone on silent or airplane mode: there will be no checking of emails, Facebook, Instagram or Snapchat feeds during rest periods.

• Track your weight: I'm not talking about the scales, I'm referring to the weight you've lifted. Have a pen and a notebook (or use your phone) to take note of what you're currently lifting. It's such a motivating way to train because you'll see and be uplifted by those strength improvements.

Choosing the right movement level for you

The main difference between the beginner and advanced programmes is in the complexity of the movements. The advanced variations require a high level of coordination and proprioception (see page 263) before you attempt them. The checklist below will help you to judge if and when you should progress to the advanced variations:

• You have not had a baby in the last six months.

• You have been weight training regularly for more than 12 months.

• You can perform 50 body weight squats, with the hips moving parallel to the knees and without a deterioration in correct alignment and form.

• You can execute 10 full push-ups with correct alignment and form.

• You can hold a full hollow body hold for 60 seconds without your lumbar (lower spine) coming off the floor.

If you can confidently tick these off (and of course pass the health questionnaire on page 104), then by all means feel free to try the advanced movements and variations. However if at any point you feel unstable in an exercise, regress it's difficulty to the beginner variation instead.

I will take this opportunity to warn you that just because the workout is labelled as 'beginner' it does not mean that it will be easy. I have put many people, that you would label as 'fit' through my beginner regimes only to see them fall to the floor in a sweaty heap. Having the fitness capacity to run a marathon does not automatically translate into the capacity to lift heavy or fast. This fitness programme is particularly demanding because it uses multijoint, compound movements to challenge your body, your coordination and raise your heart rate. I believe that if you have been weight training for less than 12 months you should not be starting with the advanced movement programme. Instead, you should start with the beginner exercises, progressively making it more difficult with the weight you lift and repetitions you manage to execute.

Track your weight: I'm not talking about the scales, I'm referring to the weight you've lifted.

Choosing the right weight for you

Choosing the right weight for you is going to be integral to an effective and yet safe workout. The weight you choose should fit the rep ranges outlined in the programme. For example, if your exercise is a kettlebell squat and the rep range is 8–10 reps, you should choose a weight that enables you to lift between 8 and 10 repetitions. You should be able to hit 8 repetitions easily, but only just get the tenth repetition. If you can barely get to 8 reps with good form, the weight is too heavy. If you can easily do 10 or more reps, the weight is too light.

If you have never lifted a weight before in your life, be conservative. Strength is relative, so what is light for some is heavy for others. For beginners, I like to suggest a 4kg kettlebell for upper body and an 8kg kettlebell for lower body. If this ends up being too light, you can always get a heavier weight later. It's better to start safe and pick up the intensity as you get better and more familiar with the programme.

I chose kettlebells because they are a practical and compact piece of equipment that enable you to perform challenging compound movements effectively. I find them more convenient than dumb-bells for at-home training. The Vertue Method does not contain advanced dynamic movements like swings or snatches, because I felt it would be irresponsible of me to suggest those highly advanced exercises. If you are interested in learning Olympic-lifting, dynamic movements, book in with a qualified personal trainer or, better yet, a strength coach. I see too many people in the gym (even advanced practitioners) performing those kinds of exercises incorrectly. Because they are fast and dynamic, there is a greater risk of injury.

HOW TO READ THE PROGRAMME

	EXERCISE	REPS	TEMPO	REST
A1	Kettlebell Goblet Box Squat (page 129)	12–15	2110	10s
	REPEAT X 3 SETS			

Exercise letters and numbers – the letters and numbers in the first column tell you the order in which to perform the exercises. The letter will represent a set and the number will obviously determine the order. For example: A1 will always be the first exercise of the first set. In the example above you will perform 3 x sets of exercise A1 before moving through the remaining A exercises. Once you've finished the A exercises you will move onto the B exercises, then the C exercises, and so on.

Exercise names – the second column represents the exercise names. These exercises and their alignment cues and instructions can be found using the page numbers as listed next to the exercise.

Reps – The third column tells you the repetitions to perform. If an exercise involves performing a movement on the left and right side of your body, the number of reps refers to the number you need to perform on each side. The number shows you the minimum and maximum requirements for each set. Remember, if you can do more than the required maximum, it's not hard enough, so go heavier with your weight.

Tempo – The fourth column instructs you on the pace of the movement. Tempo teaches you to focus on slowing or speeding up movements to create a more intense workout. From a more technical perspective, you can also increase and manipulate strength developments by slowing down the eccentric phase of a movement (the eccentric phase being the lowering portion of an exercise, where the muscle is lengthening while still being under load). Here's how to read tempo, using the example of 4010:

4 – The first number represents what is called the eccentric phase, and it gives the seconds it should take to lower into the movement. With a squat it would mean 4 seconds to lower into the bottom part of the movement.

0 – The second number represents the time I would like you to take at the bottom of the movement.

1 – The third number indicates the time it takes to get back up, or what is known as the concentric phase. In a squat it would be the time it takes to stand back up.

0 – The last number represents any pause at the top of the movement before beginning the next repetition.

Rest – It's really important that you follow my instructions on rest, and yes, it includes the time to get in position for the next exercise. If it says 10 seconds, it will usually only give you enough time to go from a squat position to the floor for a push-up position; there will be no time for selfies.

Notes
Don't forget to write some notes on how you felt during the workout, how much you lifted, and if you saw any strength improvements. Tracking progress like this is far more motivating than simply tracking visual changes.

EQUIPMENT REQUIRED

I wanted to design a programme that was accessible for those of you who can't make it to the gym and are training from home. While I love the gym and couldn't picture my life without barbells and squat racks, I also adamantly believe that you can achieve a strong, fit and healthy body with minimal equipment. Here is what you will need.

Lift
1 x light kettlebell (for upper body lifts)
1 x heavy kettlebell (for lower body lifts)
1 x yoga mat (not a fitness or Pilates mat as they are too thick and squidgy)
1 x large looped resistance band
1 x bench, block or sturdy chair

Lengthen
1 x tennis ball (or mobility ball)

Accessories
1 x water bottle (glass or aluminum)
1 x towel
1 x stopwatch (to time rests – of course you can use your phone but have it on airplane mode so that you're not disturbed)

Optional
1 x pull-up bar (for my advanced crew who are training in a gym or have a pull-up bar at home)

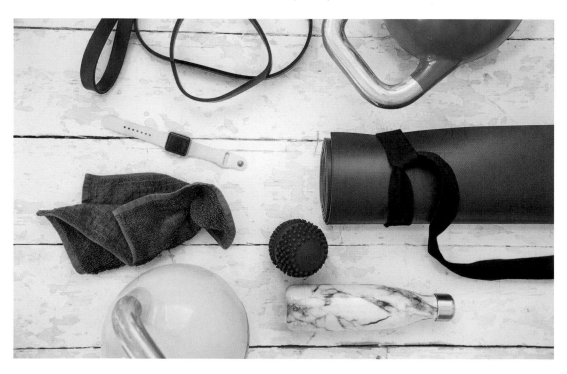

WARM UP

If you're like me, you'll have spent many a workout NOT warming up. Not only is this stupid, as it increases the risk of injury, but it also eliminates your ability to get into the focused zone of training; increasing body and breath awareness is paramount for an effective workout.

This warm up doesn't change, so once you learn it you can use it for good. It contains specific exercises to help activate important stabilisers, as well as dynamic stretches that will mobilise the joints to promote full range of motion without reducing the muscles' output capability.

	EXERCISE	REPS
W1	Belly Breathing (page 112)	10 breaths
W2 L & R	Knee Hug to Twist (page 113)	10
W3	Glute Bridge (page 114)	10
W4 L & R	Single Leg Glute Bridge (page 115)	10
W5	Quadrupled Belly Breathing (page 116)	5 breaths
W6 L & R	Bird Dog (page 117)	10
W7 L & R	Hip to Heel Thoracic Opening (page 118)	5 breaths
W8 L & R	Downdog Walks (page 119)	5 steps
W9	Caterpillar to Plank (page 120)	5
W10	Alternating Yoga Lunge (page 121)	5
W11	Alternating Step-throughs (page 122)	10
W12	Bear Crawl (page 123)	10 steps
W13	Wall Slides (page 124)	8
W14 L & R	X Band Alternating Side Steps (page 125)	10
W15	Banded Squats (page 126)	20
W16 L & R	Banded Crab Walk (page 127)	10

WU1 BELLY BREATHING

1.
Begin lying on your back with your knees bent and your feet placed just over hip distance apart. Place the left hand on the belly, right hand on the heart.

2.
Take a deep breath and relax your entire body from the head down to the toes.

3.
Inhale and feel the lower ribs rise and expand.

4.
Exhale and feel the ribs compress.

5.
Pause before you breathe in again.

6.
Repeat as directed.

Key alignment cues
Keep checking in to make sure that your neck and shoulders are relaxed.

Purpose
To relax and generate concentration as well as reminding the body to breathe out (and in). Although this pose won't warm you up, it will give you a chance to relax and check in with the body. Body and breath awareness is a really important part of training that is often overlooked. This will also begin to remind you of proper rib cage alignment.

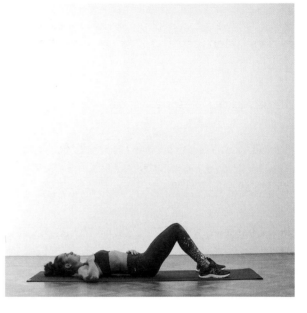

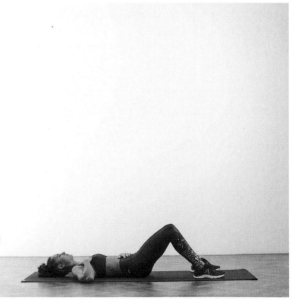

WU2 KNEE HUG TO TWIST

1.
From a reclined position, hug the left knee into the chest, interlacing your fingers around the knee.

2.
Pull the knee gently towards your armpit and hold.

3.
Take the knee across the body towards the floor as you reach your arm in the opposite direction, entering into a reclined twist.

4.
Repeat the sequence with the right knee.

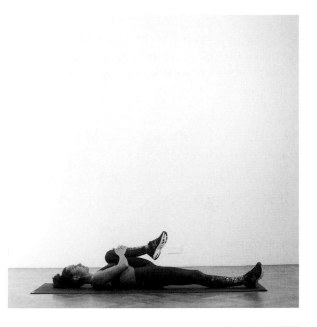

Key alignment cues
Keep your shoulders relaxed all the way through this movement. Don't force your knee to the floor if it doesn't want to go there; move mindfully and allow the body to release into the twist with the breath.

Purpose
Twists have many benefits. Aside from stretching the muscles of the back, chest, shoulder and hip, a spinal twist can also help to mobilise the spine, and even massage and stimulate the digestive organs.

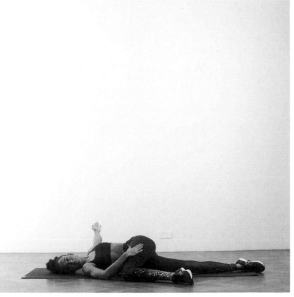

WU3 GLUTE BRIDGE

1.
From the reclined position, bend your knees and place the feet hip distance apart and flat on the floor.

2.
Begin to tuck your tail bone so that your hips raise off the floor, followed by your spinal vertebrae.

3.
Lift the hips as high as you can while squeezing your glutes.

4.
Return to the starting position, lowering the spine one vertebra at a time.

5.
Repeat as directed.

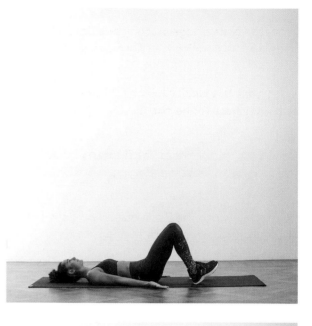

Key alignment cues
Ensure that your glutes are dominating this movement. Put your mind into the gluteal muscles and consciously squeeze them as you lift the hips. To ensure it's not your lower back doing the work, tuck your tailbone. If you don't feel your glutes, move your heels further forward.

Purpose
To switch on the glutes, of course.

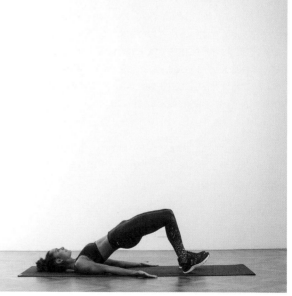

WU4 SINGLE LEG GLUTE BRIDGE

1.
From the glute bridge starting position, raise
your left leg, bending it in towards the chest.

2.
Using your left hand, grab hold of the left knee
to hold it close to the chest.

3.
Drive the right heel into the floor to lift the hips
in an explosive movement.

4.
Lower the hips to the floor, maintaining the hold
of the left leg.

5.
Repeat as directed, then switch sides.

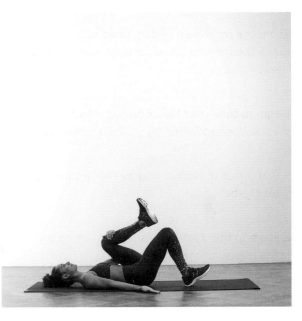

Key alignment cues
Ensure that your glutes are dominating this
movement. Put your mind into the gluteal muscles
and consciously squeeze them as you lift the
hips. By holding your knee close to your chest,
you allow the pelvis to be in a better position for
maximal glute activation.

Purpose
It will really help to activate hamstrings and glutes,
as well as waking up a little bit of contralateral
stability (stability from left to right).

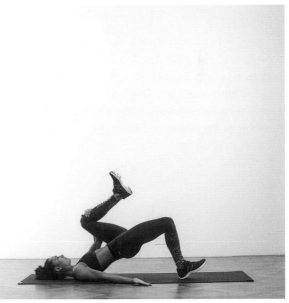

WU5 QUADRUPLED BELLY BREATHING

1.
Rock into an all-fours position, adjusting your hands shoulder distance apart, as well as your knees hip distance apart.

2.
Begin to push the floor away from you as you drop the head, pulling the ribs in deeply towards the spine.

3.
Hold the out breath for 1 second.

4.
Repeat from a relaxed position.

Key alignment cues
The breath is the most important part of this exercise. Ensure that you're pressing the floor away and that the shoulder blades don't pop out towards the ceiling. They should be flat against the back, spreading away from the spine.

Purpose
This exercise is designed to teach you correct breath awareness and ribcage/thoracic alignment. It will also activate your serratus and deactivate your latissimus dorsi (overactive lats can very often cause issues with spinal alignment as well as internal rotation).

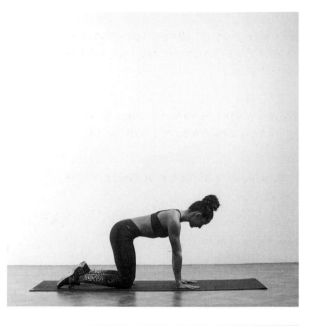

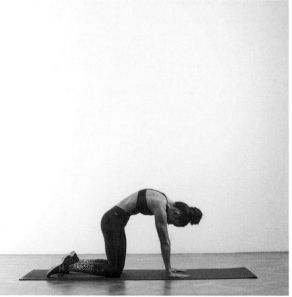

WU6 BIRD DOG

1.
Remaining in your all-fours position, begin to extend the left arm and right leg – it will require some balance.

2.
As you exhale, bend the extended arm and leg, allowing the elbow to meet the knee.

3.
Extend again and repeat as directed, then switch sides.

Key alignment cues
Don't let your spine sag as you extend. There will be a temptation to lift the hip of the extended hip, as well as a bending of the lower back. Keep your core active by drawing in the stomach, while also ensuring the pelvis remains square and flat.

Purpose
A great exercise to generate awareness of contralateral stability (stabilising the left and right sides of the body).

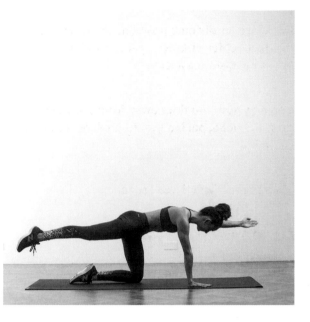

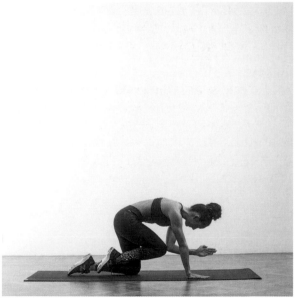

WU7 HIP TO HEEL THORACIC OPENING

1.
In the all-fours position, place the right hand onto the left shoulder.

2.
Press the hips back to the heels and keep them there.

3.
Exhale, lifting the elbow up towards the ceiling.

4.
Inhale, taking the elbow back down. Repeat as directed, then switch sides.

Key alignment cues
Try to think of lifting and twisting the whole torso rather than just moving your elbow up and down. As well, aim to keep the pelvis still to allow the stretches and mobilisation to occur within the thoracic region.

Purpose
An awesome thoracic mobiliser – an area that can get particularly tight working behind a desk all day.

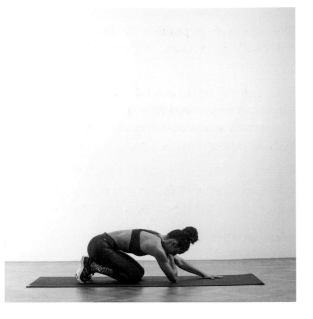

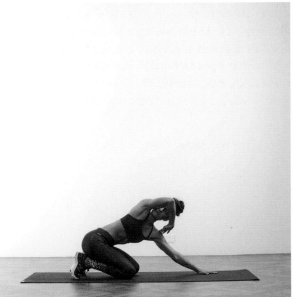

WU8 DOWNDOG WALKS

1.
From the all-fours position, lift the knees and press back into a downward facing dog.

2.
The hands will be shoulder distance apart, feet hip distance apart and your spine will be long. Try to make an upside-down V shape with your body, bending from the hips.

3.
Walk your downward facing dog position on the spot by straightening one leg, bending the other.

4.
Repeat as directed, alternating sides.

Key alignment cues
Downward facing dog pose is literally your enemy if your hamstrings and/or shoulders are tight – bending both knees will take the pressure off the shoulders that is caused by the resistance from the hamstrings and hips. Prioritise a straight and open spine here, rather than straight legs. Also be sure to keep the lower ribs pulled in.

Purpose
To release the hamstrings, calves and thoracic spine.

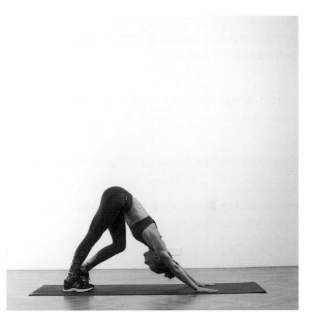

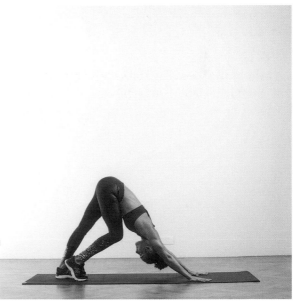

WU9 CATERPILLAR TO PLANK

1.
Begin in a standing position at the back of
your mat.

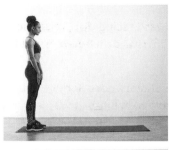

2.
Inhale, bend forward and walk your hands
out into the push-up position.

3.
Exhale, hold here.

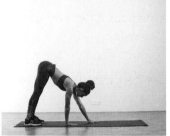

4.
Inhale, walk the hands back to the feet.

5.
Exhale, standing up, and repeat as directed.

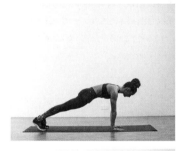

Key alignment cues
Make sure you move with the breath. Move
dynamically with concentration. Don't let the hips
sag low in your push-up position.

Purpose
This will begin to lift your heart rate while also
switching on key core stabilisers.

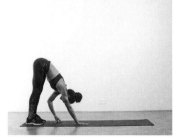

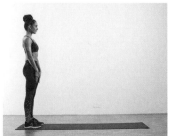

WU10 ALTERNATING YOGA LUNGE

1.
From downward facing dog, raise the left leg and swing it forward, in between your hands.

2.
Brace through your core and lift your arms and body up into a high lunge, while leaning forwards slightly.

3.
Place the hands back down and step into downward facing dog.

4.
Repeat as directed, alternating sides.

Key alignment cues
In the lunge, ensure that you stack the ankle directly under the knee. Avoid letting the knee drop forward over the toes, and do not let the heel lift off the floor.

Purpose
Dynamic moving lunges help to stretch and mobilise the hips.

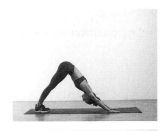

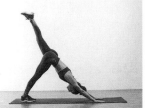

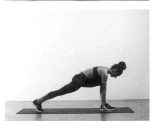

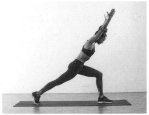

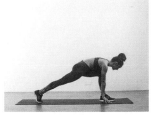

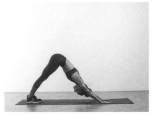

WU11 ALTERNATING STEP-THROUGHS

1.
From a downward-facing dog position, step the right leg forward to the outside of the right hand.

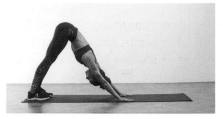

2.
Take the right hand off the floor and lift your back left leg, quickly bringing it forward.

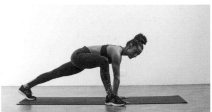

3.
Without letting the left leg touch the floor, bring the left foot through the space between the left hand and right foot.

4.
Fully extend your left leg. (It will feel like you're playing an awkward game of Twister.)

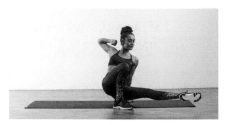

5.
Pull the left leg back, replace the right hand down on the ground and land back in a downward-facing dog position.

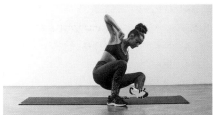

6.
Repeat as directed, alternating sides.

Key alignment cues
Try to avoid letting your lifted leg touch the floor. This will really help to activate your core.

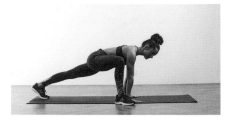

Purpose
This exercise really builds heat. If you're not sweating even a little after performing this you're either doing it wrong, or you are a part of a breakdancing troupe. It works the whole body, while also really working the internal obliques.

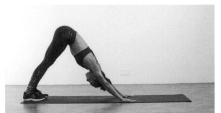

WU12 BEAR CRAWL

1.
Start in an all-fours position, with your hands shoulder distance apart and your knees hip distance apart. Raise the knees a centimetre off the floor.

2.
In a crawling motion, step the right hand an inch forward as you step the left foot an inch forward. Do not let your knees touch the floor.

3.
Repeat with the opposite side, to form a crawl movement.

4.
Move to the top of the mat in this way, and then towards the back of the mat in this way.

5.
Repeat as directed.

Key alignment cues
Don't let the knees touch the floor and try to maintain perfect alignment of the spine (no sagging through the belly).

Purpose
To improve proprioception (see Glossary, page 263) as well as bring awareness to contralateral stability. It will also strengthen the core and key spinal stabilisers.

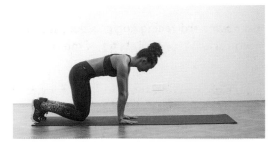
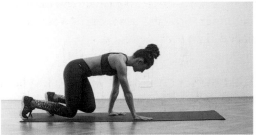
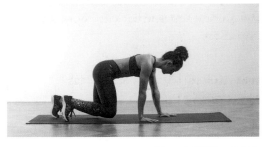
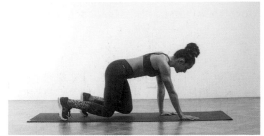
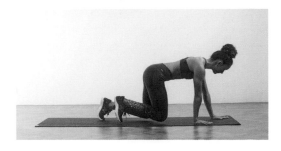

WU13 WALL SLIDES

1.
Stand facing a wall with your forearms against
the wall at a 90-degree angle.

2.
Pull the ribcage in tight and push the spine in
between the shoulder blades away from the wall
so that your shoulder blades spread away from
the midline.

3.
Begin to slowly extend your arms upward in a
Y shape.

4.
Go as far as you can without extending the spine
or lifting your elbows off the wall.

5.
Return to the start position and repeat as
directed.

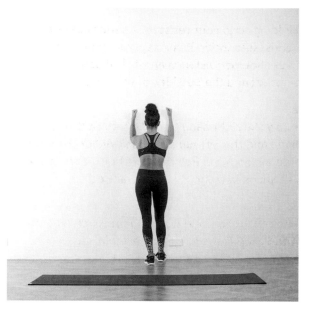

Key alignment cues
The ribs need to stay drawn throughout the entire
movement.

Purpose
To activate the serratus and relax the latissimus
dorsi.

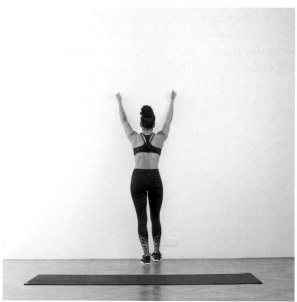

The Workouts

WU14 X BAND ALTERNATING SIDE STEPS

1.
Holding onto your resistance band with both hands, step inside it and separate your feet just over shoulder distance apart. The band should be tight around the outsides of your feet.

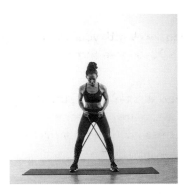

2.
Allow the right hand to pull on the left side of the band and the left hand to take hold of the right side of the band. Pull tight. It should form an 'X'-like shape in front of your lower body.

3.
Keep the resistance tight and take a step to the right. Step the left foot in very slightly.

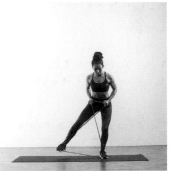

4.
Repeat as directed, alternating sides.

Key alignment cues
Keep the spine neutral, while hinging from the hips. Ensure that you lead with the knee, rather than just the foot. This will encourage the glutes to switch on.

Purpose
It really helps to switch the gluteus medius on, and is one of my favourite glute exercises.

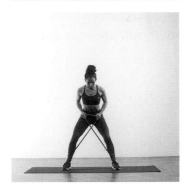

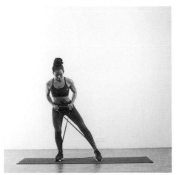

WU15 BANDED SQUAT

1.
Start with your feet shoulder width apart.

2.
Using your resistance band, make a loop in it, twisting the ends, then bring them together to form a smaller, doubled circle.

3.
Step into the circle and place the band just above the knees.

4.
Bend your knees, push your hips back, but aim to keep your chest lifted.

5.
Inhale as you continue to lower the hips as much as possible, while keeping your spine in a neutral position. Resist the band with your knees.

6.
Exhale and quickly push through the heels to stand up, returning to the starting position.

7.
Repeat as directed.

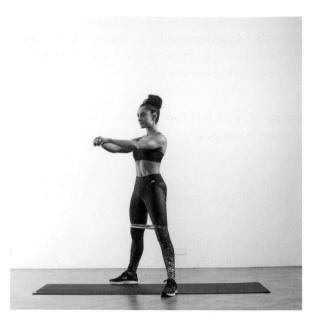

Key alignment cues
Do not let your knees drop inwardly as you lower into the squat. Keep them pushing outwards (this will teach your glutes to stay active in a squat). Don't let your heels lift off the floor at any stage of the squat. Don't let your lower back round.

Purpose
Squatting is a human movement required not just for practical things like getting in and out of chairs, but it also supports our digestive system by massaging our ascending and descending colons. It is also a great lower body exercise that in addition to glute and thighs also works your core (spinal stabilisers). The band around the knees forces the glutes to switch on.

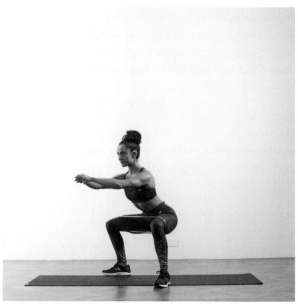

WU16 BANDED CRAB WALK

1.
From that squatted position, begin to take a step to the right, creating extra tension on the band, pushing the knees outward.

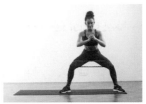

2.
Follow with the left foot, keeping the hips low and the knees pushing outward.

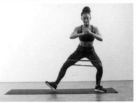

3.
Repeat this step again, stepping to the right again, with the left foot following shortly afterwards.

4.
Repeat 5 steps on the right, then swap to repeat 5 steps on the left. Continue until you've done 10 on both sides.

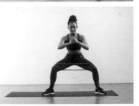

Key alignment cues
Do not let your knees drop inwardly as you crab walk. Keep them pushing outwardly (this will teach your glutes to stay active). Land with the heels down first and keep the chest lifted; avoid flaring through the ribcage but maintain a strong torso that isn't rounded.

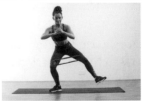

Purpose
Another exercise to really wake up your glutes, as well as encourage spinal stabilisation through weight transfer.

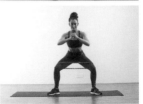

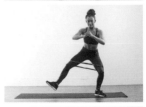

WE ARE READY TO TRAIN!
Have you:
Got all your equipment laid out?
Got water?

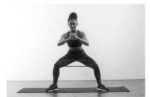

BEGINNERS – VM WORKOUT 1

	EXERCISE	REPS	TEMPO	REST
A1	Kettlebell Goblet Box Squat (page 129)	12–15	2110	10s
A2	Elevated Hands Close Grip Push-up (page 130)	10–12	3010	10s
A3 L & R	Straight Arm Reverse Kettlebell Lunge (page 131)	12–15	2010	10s
A4 L & R	Chair/ Bench Single Arm Row (page 132)	10–12	2010	30s
REPEAT X 3 SETS				
B1 L & R	Kettlebell Single Leg Glute Bridge (page 133)	12–15	1010	10s
B2 L & R	Side Lying Hip Raise (page 134)	15	1010	30s
REPEAT X 3 SETS				
C1	Reverse Crunch (page 135)	15	1010	10s
C2	Kettlebell Crunch (page 136)	15	1010	10s
C3	Mountain Climbers (page 137)	30	1010	10s
C4	Cobra Lifts (page 138)	10	1210	30s
REPEAT X 3 SETS				

IF YOU'RE GOING TO THE GYM DON'T FORGET TO TAKE A PHOTO OF THIS PAGE WITH YOUR PHONE SO YOU CAN DO THE WORKOUT.

A1 KETTLEBELL GOBLET BOX SQUAT

1.
Begin with a wide stance, slightly wider than the shoulders. Slightly turn out the toes (roughly 30 degrees).

2.
Take a deep breath, bend at the knees and begin to drop your hips backwards towards a chair/bench, moving into a squatting position. Keep your chest proud as you lower into the squat without flaring at the ribs. Sit down onto the chair while maintaining integrity of a long spine (you will want to round your back but it's important that you keep a healthy arch in your lower back at the bottom of the squat).

3.
Keep your chest lifted and rise up out of the squat with a tall spine, squeezing your glutes at the top of the movement.

Key alignment cues
Drive the outer edge of your heel into the floor as you rise out of the squat. This should stop your knees from dropping into the centre.

Main muscles worked
Quads and glutes. The squat is a knee-dominant movement and therefore places emphasis on the quads, but with a slightly wider stance and specific alignment cues it also works glutes (at the bottom) and erectors (which are back muscles). The squat also helps develop core stability by holding the spine in a neutral position under load.

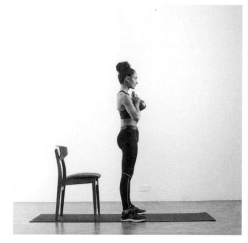

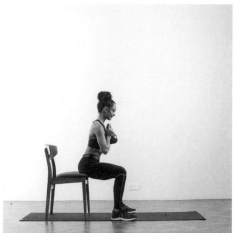

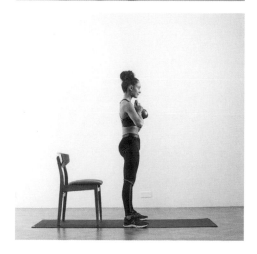

A2 ELEVATED HANDS CLOSE GRIP PUSH-UP

1.
Place your hands onto the chair/bench in a push-up position. Make sure your wrists are stacked just under the shoulders. Spread your thumbs wide and then bring them together to touch – this will be the distance of your close grip.

2.
Walk your feet backwards so that your hips can extend, allowing for correct spinal and pelvic alignment. You should be in one long line from head to feet.

3.
Take a deep breath in, bend at the elbows and begin to lower the chest towards the chair. Keep the elbows close as you lower towards the chair.

4.
Go as deep as possible into the push-up while maintaining integrity to the spine and pelvis.

5.
Press back up to the starting position without letting your shoulders rise up the ears.

Key alignment cues
The elbows should shave the sides of your body as you rise up and drop into the push-up. Do not let your upper shoulders take over the movement; try to keep them relaxed.

Main muscles worked
Triceps. The close grip push-up is a favourite variation for me because of the loading it puts on the triceps. Most women don't want large pectorals so this is the variation I emphasise for my female clients. Men also tend to neglect their tricep development and work on growing a massive chest and biceps (there is nothing wrong with that, but ladies love triceps too).

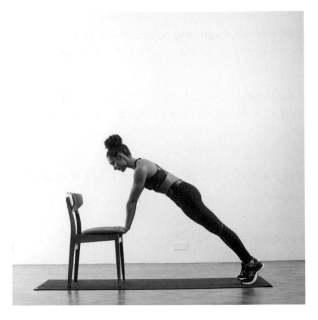

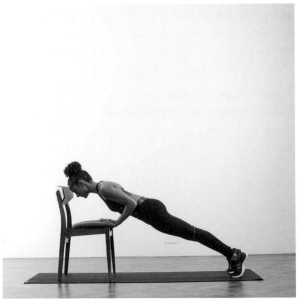

A3 STRAIGHT ARM REVERSE KETTLEBELL LUNGE

1.
Begin from a standing position with the kettlebell in the right hand, with your left hand on your hip.

2.
Take a giant step back with the left leg, into a long lunge until your right leg comes into a 90-degree angle.

3.
Press through the heel and return to a standing position.

4.
Repeat as directed, then switch sides.

Key alignment cues
Keep the spine neutral at all times and avoid letting your lower belly relax. Keep it lightly pulled inward. To really activate your glutes in this movement, ensure that your ankle does not go beyond the toes. Press through the heel to stand up out of the lunge.

Main muscles worked
This is a knee-dominant movement, so technically speaking it really works your quads. However, I tweak all my lunges by making them extra-long in stance so that my hamstrings and glutes have to fire to get me out of the deep lunge.

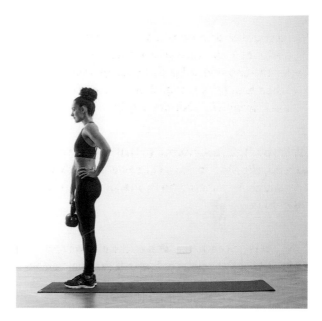

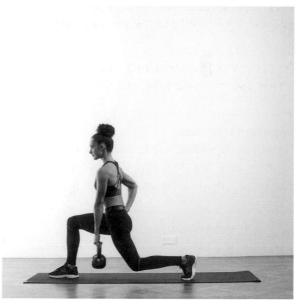

A4 CHAIR/BENCH SUPPORTED SINGLE ARM ROW

1.
Place the kettlebell on your chair/bench.

2.
Place the right leg on top of the end of the chair, bend forward from the hips until your upper body is parallel to the floor, and place your right hand on the other end of the chair for support.

3.
Using the right hand, pick up the kettlebell and hold it while keeping your lower back straight and belly button hugging towards the spine. This is the starting position.

4.
Exhale and pull the kettlebell straight up to the side of your chest, keeping your upper arm close to your side and keeping the body still (no movement through the torso).

5.
Inhale and return to the starting position.

Key alignment cues
The spine must stay neutral; do not let your upper back round. You want to lead the movement from your shoulder blade rather than your arm.

Main muscles worked
Middle back, lower trapezius, some latissimus dorsi as well as deep anti-rotational core muscles.

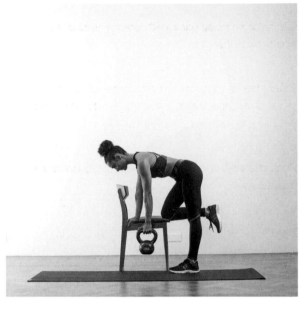

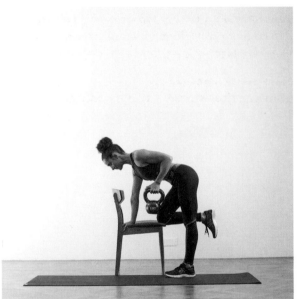

B1 KETTLEBELL SINGLE LEG GLUTE BRIDGE

1.
Come onto your back with your knees bent and feet together.

2.
Raise the left leg off the floor, bending the knee in towards your chest. Place the kettlebell over your right hip.

3.
Push the right heel into the floor and drive your hips up towards the ceiling.

4.
Return to the starting position.

5.
Repeat as directed, then switch sides.

Key alignment cues
Keep the raised knee close towards your chest to ensure that your tail bone remains tucked. Keep your shoulders relaxed.

Main muscles worked
Glutes and hamstrings – all the good stuff.

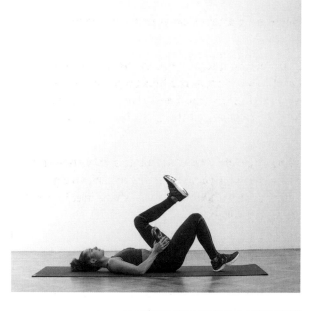

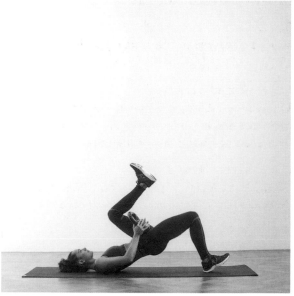

B2 SIDE LYING HIP RAISE

1.
Roll over onto your right side, placing your right elbow underneath your right shoulder. Ensure your palm is down and the forearm and wrist are in line with the elbow. Bend your right leg at a 45-degree angle. Ensure that your hip and ankle are in alignment. Straighten the left leg and lift the left ankle off the floor. This is your starting position.

2.
Push into the right knee (with some support from the elbow), lifting your hips off the floor.

3.
Lower back down to the starting position for repetition.

4.
Repeat as directed, then switch sides.

Key alignment cues
Keep your core tight; imagine wearing a corset. There should be no movement between the ribs and hips.

Main muscles worked
This is such a glute burner, and of course your shoulder will feel a little worked as well. If you feel it in your back, it usually means that your erectors and quadratus lumborum (back muscles) are trying to do the work, rather than the glutes.

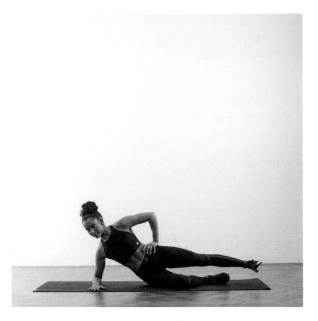

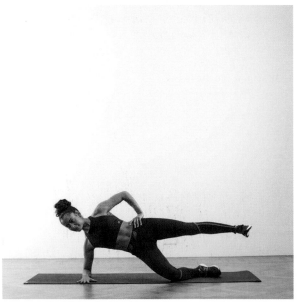

C1 REVERSE CRUNCH

1.
Come onto your back with your knees bent
and feet together.

2.
Pull the knees towards the head, raising the
hips off the floor.

3.
Return to the starting position.

Key alignment cues
Try to avoid pushing hard into the ground with
your hands. They should just lightly support. Avoid
swinging the legs; the movement needs to come
from the contraction of the lower abs, rather than
the momentum of swinging legs.

Main muscles worked
If performed correctly, this exercise really helps
to recruit the lower abs.

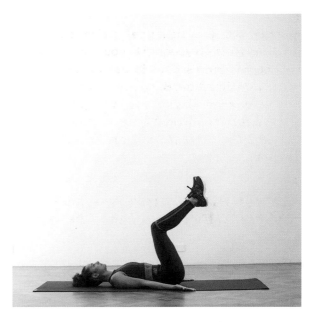

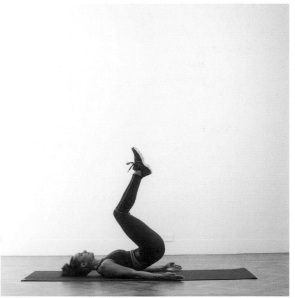

C2 KETTLEBELL CRUNCH

1.
Bring your kettlebell onto your chest. Come onto your back with your knees bent and feet hip distance apart.

2.
Straighten your arms up towards the ceiling, keeping your neck long and shoulders relaxed.

3.
Begin to curl the spine off the floor, until your middle back only lifts off, pressing the kettlebell up towards the ceiling.

4.
Lower back down with control, rolling down one vertebra at a time to the floor.

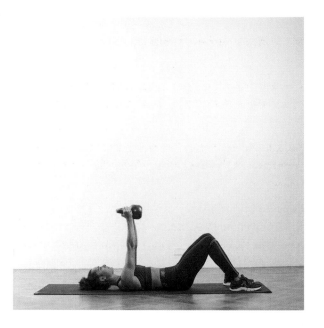

Key alignment cues
Draw the lower belly in before you move. Keep the neck and shoulders as relaxed as possible. Use your abs.

Main muscles worked
Rectus abdominus (six-pack) as well as deeper core.

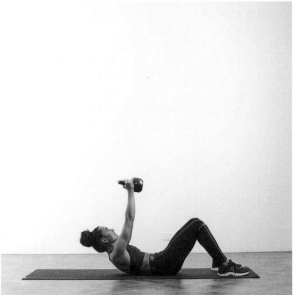

C3 MOUNTAIN CLIMBERS

1.
Move into a push-up position.

2.
Quickly bring the right knee towards the back of the right elbow (try to make them touch).

3.
In a fast, almost jumping motion, switch legs and try to touch the back of the left elbow with your left knee.

4.
Repeat as quickly as possible.

Key alignment cues
Suck your belly in during the entire movement. Keep it fast and dynamic and keep your hips at a neutral height, not higher or lower than the shoulders.

Main muscles worked
All-out everything kind of move, but if performed correctly, you will feel this in your lower abs too.

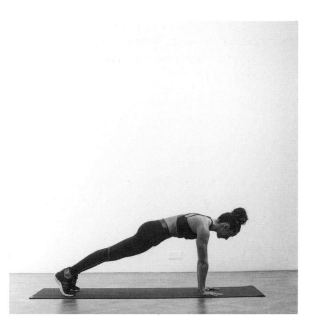

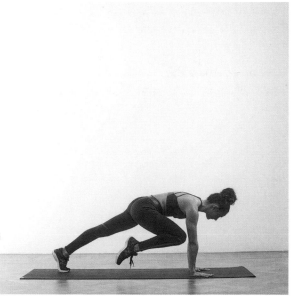

C4 COBRA LIFTS

1.
Come to lie on your stomach, placing your wrists underneath the shoulders.

2.
Exhale to lift your chest off the floor.

3.
Inhale and return to the starting position.

Key alignment cues
Keep your belly drawn inwardly, while pushing your pubic bone into the floor. Aim to keep the lower back as lengthened as possible.

Main muscles worked
Upper and middle back muscles (anti-laptop, smartphone and desktop muscles).

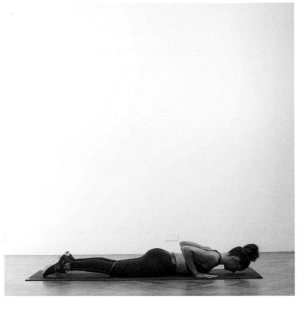

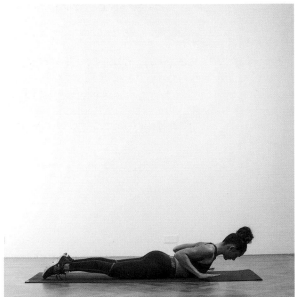

BEGINNERS – VM WORKOUT 2

	EXERCISE	REPS	TEMPO	REST
A1	Shoulder Elevated Kettlebell Hip Thrust (page 140)	12–15	2110	10s
A2	Elevated Hands Wide Grip Push-up (page 141)	10–12	3010	10s
A3	Back Foot Raised Lunge (page 142)	12–15	2010	10s
A4	Kettlebell Pullover in Deadbug Position (page 143)	6–8	5010	30s
	REPEAT X 3 SETS			
B1 L & R	Eccentric Single Leg Squat (page 144)	12–15	1010	10s
B2 L & R	Banded Kickback (page 145)	20	1010	30s
	REPEAT X 3 SETS			
C1	Alternating Step Up (page 146)	15	1010	10s
C2	Seated Band Abduction (page 147)	30	1010	10s
	REPEAT X 3 SETS			
D1 L & R	Forearm Side Plank Hip Raise (page 148)	10	1010	20s
D2	Bicycle (page 149)	30	1010	10s
D3	Cross Body Mountain Climbers (page 150)	30	1010	20s

IF YOU'RE GOING TO THE GYM DON'T FORGET TO TAKE A PHOTO OF THIS PAGE WITH YOUR PHONE SO YOU CAN DO THE WORKOUT.

A1 SHOULDER ELEVATED KETTLEBELL HIP THRUST

1.
Begin by sitting with the backs of your shoulders up against your chair/bench. Place the kettlebell on top or your hips.

2.
Pushing through your heels, lift your hips towards the ceiling until they align with the height of your shoulders. Squeeze your glutes.

3.
Lower your hips back down towards the floor (without touching) then repeat.

Key alignment cues
Dig your heels into the floor, draw your tummy in and tuck your tail bone as though you wanted to push your pubic bone towards the ceiling. Watch out for bending of the lower back, try to lengthen out the lower spine.

Main muscles worked
Glutes, baby, this should be all about the glutes. Some hamstring and very minimal quads.

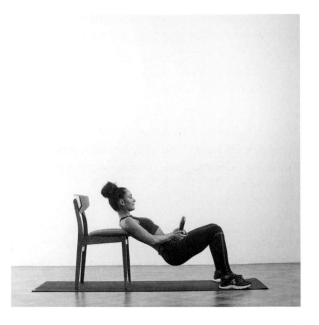

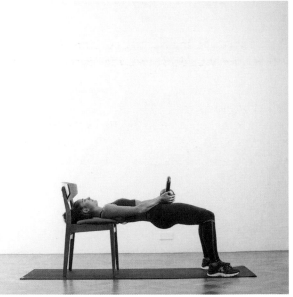

A2 ELEVATED HANDS WIDE GRIP PUSH-UP

1.
Place your hands on the chair/bench in a push-up position. Make sure your wrists are stacked just under the shoulders. Take the hands just over shoulder distance apart.

2.
Walk your feet backwards so that your hips can extend, allowing for correct spinal and pelvic alignment. You should be in one long line from head to feet.

3.
Take a deep breath in, bend at the elbows and begin to lower the chest towards the chair. Keep the elbows close as you lower towards the chair.

4.
Go as deep as possible into the push-up while maintaining integrity to the spine and pelvis.

5.
Press back up to the starting position without letting your shoulders rise up the ears.

Key alignment cues
Avoid letting your hips sag towards the floor. Keep the neck long, try to avoid letting the upper trapezius take over, keeping the shoulders away from the ears.

Main muscles worked
Pectorals.

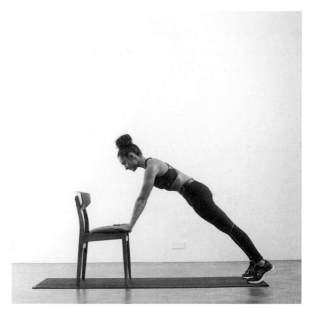

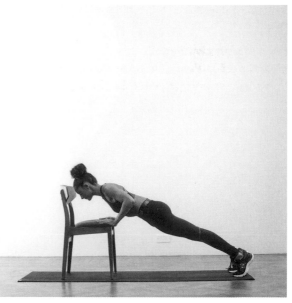

A3 BACK FOOT RAISED LUNGE

1.
Facing away from your block or chair, shift the weight onto the right side and lift the left leg up onto the bench/block or chair behind you. Place your foot on the bench with your shoelaces facing down.

2.
Hop your front leg a little further forward so you are in a fairly long stance.

3.
Bend both knees and begin to lower the back knee towards the floor.

4.
Return to the top of the lunge quickly.

Key alignment cues
Avoid overarching the lower back when you get to the bottom of the lunge. If you feel tight in the quad of the raised leg, bend the knee more. Keep your weight in the heel of the front foot.

Main muscles worked
Glutes and hamstrings. It's also great for increasing flexibility.

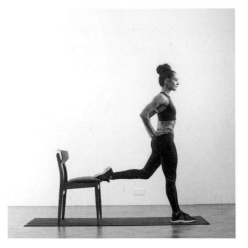

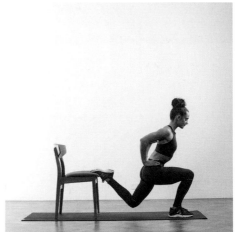

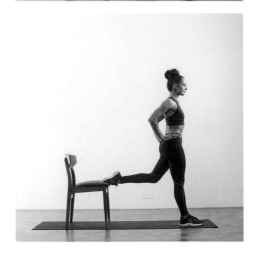

A4 KETTLEBELL PULLOVER IN DEADBUG POSITION

1.
Holding your kettlebell by the horns, come onto your back in a table-top position with your arms straight above your chest.

2.
Keeping the ribs in and belly button drawn towards the spine, begin to extend the kettlebell above your head.

3.
Bring the kettlebell back to the starting position and repeat.

Key alignment cues
Avoid letting your lower back come off the floor, keep your ribs flat and your neck relaxed.

Main muscles worked
The lats and abs.

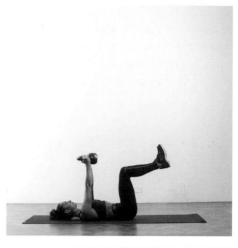

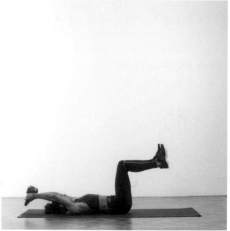

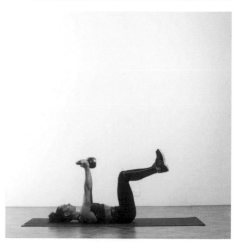

B1 ECCENTRIC SINGLE LEG SQUAT (to the chair or bench)

1.
Stand facing away from the chair/bench. Placing your hands on your hips, raise the left leg.

2.
Keeping your chest tall, push your hips back and start to squat towards the chair behind you.

3.
Sit all the way down, place your left foot down and use it to help you return to the starting position.

4.
Repeat as directed, then switch sides.

Key alignment cues
It will be really tempting to let your supporting heel come off the floor as you lower into the squat. Push the hips backwards and try to imitate the same stature that you would have in a regular squat.

Main muscles worked
Glutes and quads.

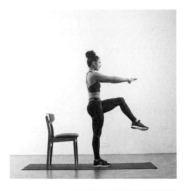

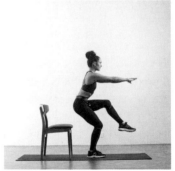

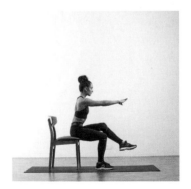

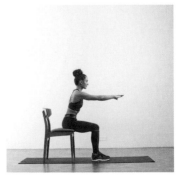

B2 BANDED KICKBACK

1.
Come into an all-fours position inside the band, with one edge of the band hooked around the thumbs.

2.
Hook the other side of the band around your right heel and extend the right leg, squeezing the glute against the resistance.

3.
Return to centre and repeat as directed, then switch sides.

Key alignment cues
Avoid letting the hips lift or tilt and maintain a neutral spine. You will want to bend the lower back as you extend your leg, but it's important to use your core and shoulder stability to stop this from happening, to fully work your glutes.

Main muscles worked
Glutes and quads.

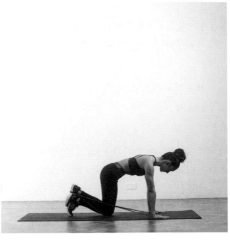

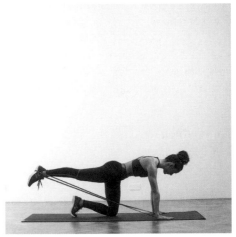

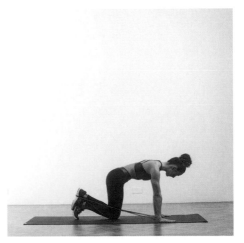

C1 ALTERNATING STEP UP

1.
Facing your chair/bench, place the right foot on top of it. Place your hands on your hips and lift through the chest.

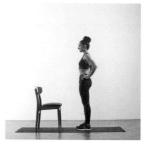

2.
Drive through the heel of your right leg (trying your best not to push off the left) and step up onto the chair.

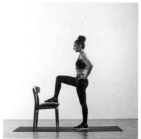

3.
Once you're up, place the left foot on the chair and step your right foot down to the ground.

4.
Keep that left leg on the bench and step up with the left leg.

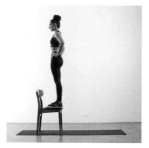

5.
Place the right foot down and step off with the left.

6.
Repeat this movement dynamically, alternating legs.

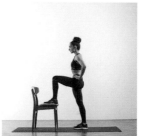

Key alignment cues
Make this more about your glutes, by leaning forwards slightly (to create a stretch in the hamstrings and glutes) and driving through the heel to stand up.

Main muscles worked
Glutes and quads.

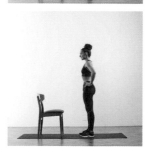

C2 SEATED BAND ABDUCTION

1.
Place the looped band around the knees
(remember to loop it twice).

2.
Sit on the edge of your chair/bench, with your
hands on your hips, chest lifted. Lean forward
slightly, pushing your hips back.

3.
Push the knees out wide against the band as
far as you can.

4.
Return to the starting position then repeat
as directed.

Key alignment cues
Avoid rounding your lower back. Keep the
chest lifted and the shoulders relaxed.

Main muscles worked
Gluteals (particularly gluteus medius).

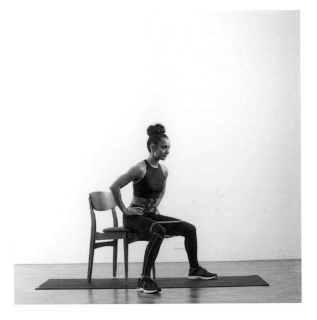

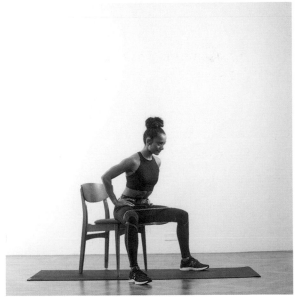

D1 FOREARM SIDE PLANK HIP RAISE

1.
Roll onto your left side, coming into a forearm side plank position.

2.
Lift your hips up and down, keeping the right hand on the hip.

3.
Repeat as directed, then switch sides.

Key alignment cues
If you feel this in your lower back, tip the top hip down slightly. Make sure your head stays in alignment with your body.

Main muscles worked
Obliques.

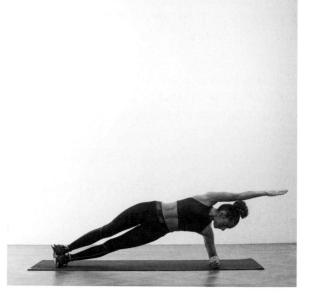

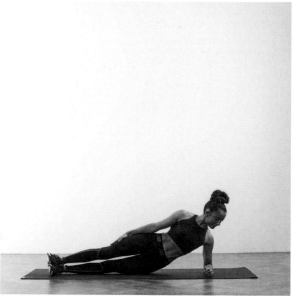

The Workouts

D2 BICYCLES

1.
Lie on your back with the knees bent up towards the ceiling.

2.
Place your fingers onto your ears, flex and rotate the upper spine by raising the upper body off the ground. Your shoulder blades should not be on the floor.

3.
Twist to bring the elbow to its opposing knee and vice versa.

4.
Repeat as directed, alternating sides.

Key alignment cues
Keep your belly button pulled inwardly towards the spine throughout the movement. Try not to let your lower back come off the floor.

Main muscles worked
Rectus abdominus (six-pack) and a little of the internal and external obliques.

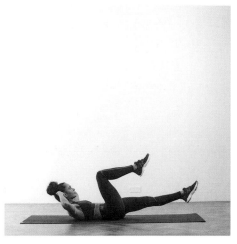

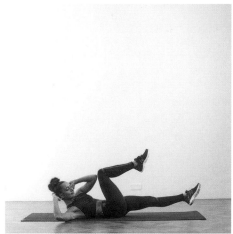

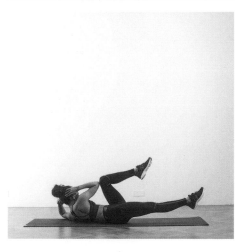

D3 CROSS BODY MOUNTAIN CLIMBERS

1.
Move into a push-up position.

2.
Quickly bring the right knee towards the back
of the left elbow (try to make them touch).

3.
In a fast, almost jumping motion, switch legs and
try to touch the back of the right elbow with your
left knee.

4.
Repeat as quickly as possible.

Key alignment cues
Suck your belly in during the entire movement.
Keep it fast and dynamic and keep your hips at
a neutral height, not higher or lower than the
shoulders.

Main muscles worked
All-out everything kind of move, but if performed
correctly, you will feel this in your lower abs and
obliques too.

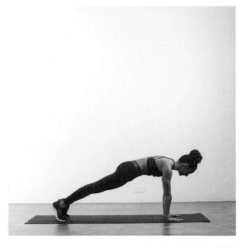

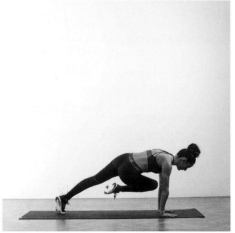

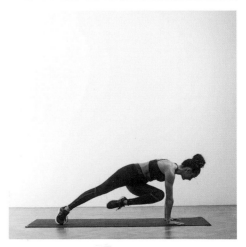

BEGINNERS – VM WORKOUT 3 (CARDIO)

	EXERCISE	REPS	REST
A1	Dynamic Alternating Step Back Lunge (page 152)	20	0s
A2	Mountain Climbers (page 153)	20	0s
A3	Alternating Squat to Side Kick (page 154)	20	0s
A4	Half Burpee (page 155)	20	0s
A5	Explosive Sumo Squat (page 156)	20	0s
A6	Shoulder Taps (page 157)	20	0s
REPEAT AS MANY ROUNDS AS POSSIBLE FOR 10 MINUTES			
B1	Bent Knee Hollow Body Hold (page 158)	45s	15s
B2	Alternating Cross Body Crunch (page 159)	45s	15s
B3	Crunches (page 160)	45s	15s
B4	Reverse Crunch to Sit Up (page 161)	45s	15s
REPEAT AS MANY ROUNDS AS POSSIBLE FOR 10 MINUTES			

IF YOU'RE GOING TO THE GYM DON'T FORGET TO TAKE A PHOTO OF THIS PAGE WITH YOUR PHONE SO YOU CAN DO THE WORKOUT.

A1 DYNAMIC ALTERNATING STEP BACK LUNGE

1.
Begin from a standing position, placing your hands on your hips.

2.
Take a giant step back with the left leg into a long lunge, until your right leg comes into a 90-degree angle.

3.
Drive through the right heel to quickly come out of the lunge.

4.
Repeat immediately on the right leg without rest, alternating as quickly as possible.

Key alignment cues
Keep the spine neutral at all times and avoid letting your lower belly relax; keep it lightly pulled inwards. To really activate your glute in this movement, ensure that your knee does not go beyond the toes. Press through the heel while coming in and out of the lunge.

Main muscles worked
A lunge is predominantly a quadriceps working movement, however because it is both dynamic and long (in stance) it should also recruit your glute and hamstrings.

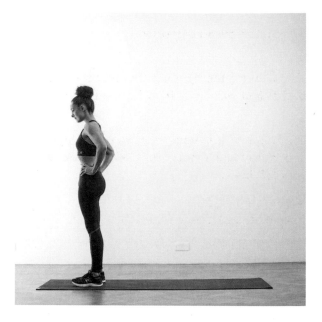

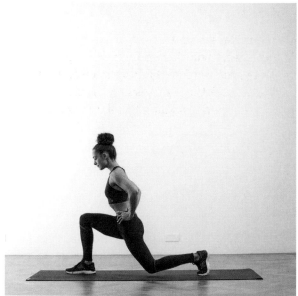

A2 MOUNTAIN CLIMBERS

1.
Move into a push-up position.

2.
Quickly bring the right knee towards the back of the right elbow (try to make them touch).

3.
In a fast, almost jumping motion, switch legs and try to touch the back of the left elbow with your left knee.

4.
Repeat as quickly as possible.

Key alignment cues
Suck your belly in during the entire movement. Keep it fast and dynamic and keep your hips at a neutral height, not higher or lower than the shoulders.

Main muscles worked
All-out everything kind of move, but if performed correctly, you will feel this in your lower abs too. It will also work the shoulders and by the twentieth repetition you will feel them burn.

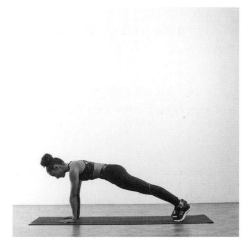

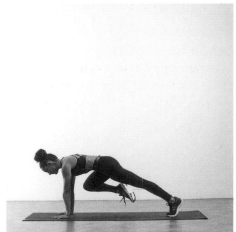

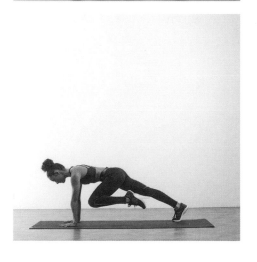

A3 ALTERNATING SQUAT TO SIDE KICK

1.
Take a squat stance (as instructed on page 126 but without the band) and move into your squat position.

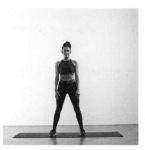

2.
As you begin to rise up and out of the squat, lean onto the left leg and side kick your right leg.

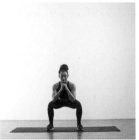

3.
Return back to the squat and prepare to kick to the left.

4.
Repeat this sequence.

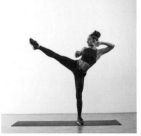

Key alignment cues
This is dynamic, but ensure that you still exercise the same neutral spine as in a usual squat. Just because it's fast, it doesn't mean it should lose all focus.

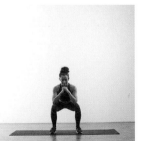

Main muscles worked
Glutes and hamstrings. It's also great for lifting the heart rate and adding some fire to the HIIT session.

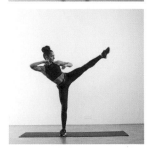

The Workouts

A4 HALF BURPEE

1.
Bend over and place your hands on the floor.

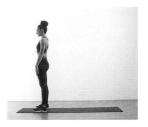

2.
Jump the feet back into a push-up position.

3.
Lower your body down to the floor.

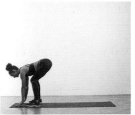

4.
Press back up to push-up position.

5.
Jump the feet back to the outsides of your hands.

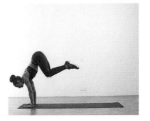

6.
Stand up quickly and repeat.

Key alignment cues
Burpees are a great exercise aerobically, but realistically they aren't teaching you anything amazing about form or correct movement patterns. As best as possible, try to maintain all the cues for push-ups and squats that I've outlined in this book so that you are staying safe throughout this movement.

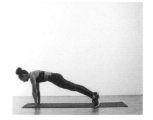

Main muscles worked
Everything. Especially the heart.

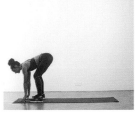

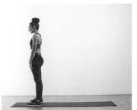

A5 EXPLOSIVE SUMO SQUAT

1.
Take your feet much wider than shoulder distance apart and bring your palms together in front of your chest.

2.
Keeping your chest lifted, drop the hips down into a squat, keeping the spine neutral.

3.
Very quickly drive back up out of the squat in an explosive movement, pushing into the heels and squeezing your glutes.

4.
Repeat moving up and down.

Key alignment cues
Maintain those squatting principles I have outlined already, but try to move quickly and dynamically. Keep your chest up at all times and do not let the spine round.

Main muscles worked
Glutes, hamstrings and adductors.

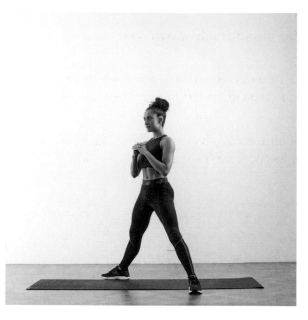

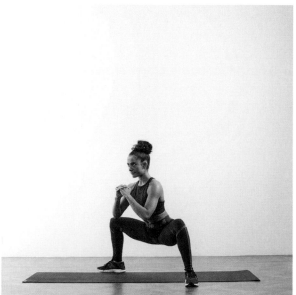

The Workouts

A6 SHOULDER TAPS

1.
Come into a push-up position.

2.
Shift the weight of your body onto the right side and tap the left hand to the right shoulder.

3.
Repeat quickly on the right side, then repeat as directed, continuing to alternate sides.

Key alignment cues
Use your anti-rotational muscles to avoid letting the hips move from side to side. Do NOT let your hips sag towards the floor.

Main muscles worked
Core and shoulder stabilisers.

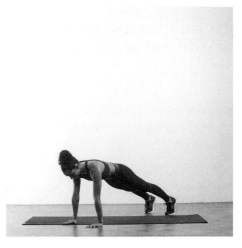

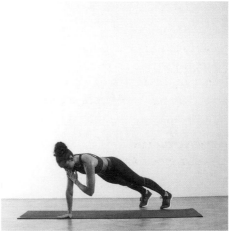

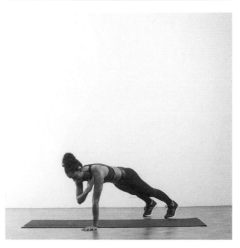

B1 BENT KNEE HOLLOW BODY HOLD

1.
Lying on your back, draw your belly button down towards the floor, and press your lower spine into the floor.

2.
Keep your abs and butt tight at all times, reach your arms towards your feet and curl your upper spine and shoulders off the floor.

3.
Slowly raise the legs off the floor, bending the knees at a 90-degree angle, making a shallow bowl shape with your body.

4.
Hold here for the time specified.

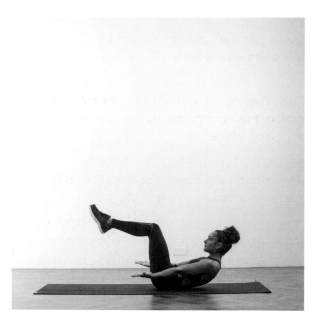

Key alignment cues
Try to maintain a bowl-like position without losing integrity of the spine. Belly stays flat and drawn inwardly.

Main muscles worked
Abdominals.

B2 ALTERNATING CROSS BODY CRUNCH

1.
Lie on your back in a starfish position
(arms and legs splayed out).

2.
Raise the left arm and right leg towards the
ceiling, touching the outside of your right foot
with your left hand.

3.
Return to the floor and repeat for the time
specified, alternating sides.

Key alignment cues
Focus on creating that same dish position that
you held during the hollow body hold, with an
emphasis on the twist.

Main muscles worked
Rectus abdominus (six-pack) and obliques.

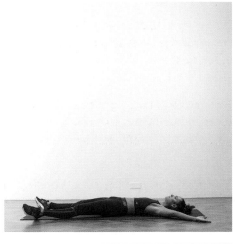

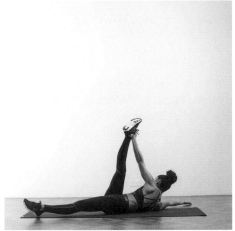

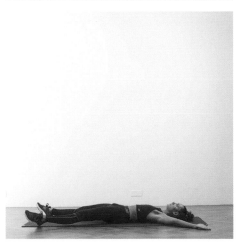

B3 CRUNCHES

1.

Lie on your back with your knees bent and feet hip distance apart. Place your fingertips lightly against the ears, with your elbows out to the sides. This will be your starting position.

2.

As you exhale, curl the spine, lifting your head, shoulders and, if possible, the back of your ribs off the floor.

3.

While inhaling, lower your body back to the starting position.

4.

Repeat.

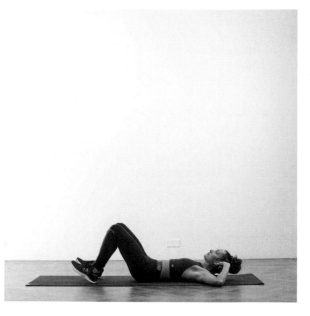

Key alignment cues

It's very tempting in a crunch to contract your neck flexors and shoulders, but this is incorrect and will only leave you feeling sore in your neck. Try to bring all your focus and attention to the abs, while relaxing your shoulders.

Main muscles worked

Rectus abdominus (six-pack) and a little of the internal and external obliques.

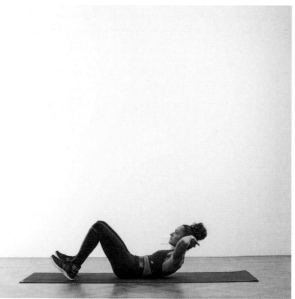

B4 REVERSE CRUNCH TO SIT-UP

1.
Come onto your back with your knees bent
and feet together, extending your arms above
your head.

2.
Draw the belly button in towards the spine, using
your core, lift the legs, hips and lower back off
the floor.

3.
Return to the starting position.

4.
Take your arms forwards, reaching towards
your knees and use your upper abs to curl your
shoulders off the floor. Continue to sit up and
raise your arms above your head.

Key alignment cues
Try to avoid pushing hard into the ground with
your hands; they should just lightly support. Avoid
swinging the legs – the movement needs to come
from the contraction of the lower abs rather than
the momentum of swinging legs.

Main muscles worked
If performed correctly this exercise really helps to
recruit the lower abs, as well as the upper rectus
abdominus.

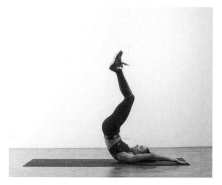

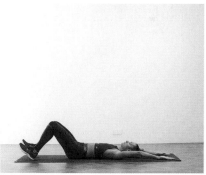

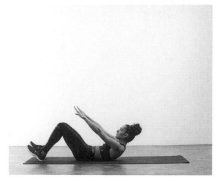

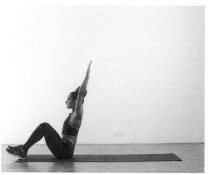

ADVANCED – VM WORKOUT 1

	EXERCISE	REPS	TEMPO	REST
A1	Kettlebell Goblet Pause Squat (page 163)	10–12	2110	10s
A2	Close Grip Push-up (page 164)	8–10	3010	10s
A3 L & R	Bent Arm Reverse Kettlebell Lunge (page 165)	12–15	2010	10s
A4 L & R	Lunge Stance Single Arm Row (page 166)	10–12	2010	30s
REPEAT X 3 SETS				
B1 L & R	Kettlebell Single Leg Glute Bridge (page 167)	12–15	1010	10s
B2 L & R	Side Lying Hip Raise (page 168)	12–15	1010	30s
REPEAT X 3 SETS				
C1	Reverse Crunch (page 169)	15	1010	10s
C2	Kettlebell Crunch (page 170)	15	1010	10s
C3	Table Top Rocks (page 171)	10	1110	10s
C4	Push-up to Bird Dog (page 172)	10	1010	30s
REPEAT X 3 SETS				

IF YOU'RE GOING TO THE GYM DON'T FORGET TO TAKE A PHOTO OF THIS PAGE WITH YOUR PHONE SO YOU CAN DO THE WORKOUT.

A1 KETTLEBELL GOBLET PAUSE SQUAT

1.
Grab the handles of your kettlebell and hold it directly under your chin resting on your chest. Begin with a wide stance, slightly wider than the shoulders. Slightly turn out the toes (roughly 30 degrees).

2.
Take a deep breath, bend at the knees and begin to drop your hips backwards, moving into a squatting position. Keep your chest proud as you lower into the squat without flaring at the ribs. Sit deep into the squat while maintaining integrity of a long spine (you will want to round your back but it's important that you keep a healthy arch in your lower back at the bottom of the squat).

3.
Pause at the depth of the squat for 1 second, while keeping your chest lifted.

4.
Rise up out of the squat with a tall spine, squeezing your glutes at the top of the movement.

Key alignment cues
Drive the outer edge of your heel into the floor as you rise out of the squat. This should stop your knees from dropping into the centre.

Main muscles worked
Quads and glutes. The squat is a knee-dominant movement and therefore places emphasis on the quads. However, with a slightly wider stance and specific alignment cues, it also works glutes (at the bottom) and erectors (which are back muscles). The squat also helps develop core stability by holding the spine in a neutral position under load.

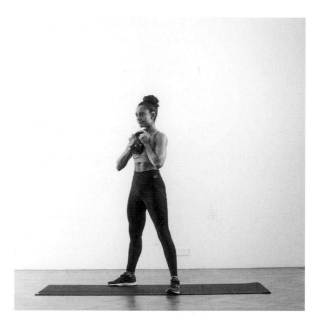

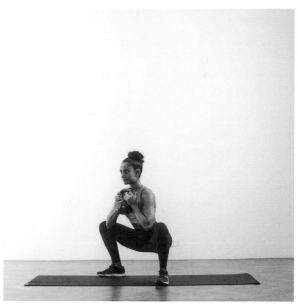

A2 CLOSE GRIP PUSH-UP

1.
Begin in a push-up position. Make sure your wrists are stacked just under the shoulders. Spread your thumbs wide and then bring them together to touch – this will be the distance of your close grip.

2.
Take a deep breath in, bend at the elbows and begin to lower the chest towards the floor, keeping the elbows close.

4.
Go as deep as possible into the push-up while maintaining integrity to the spine and pelvis.

5.
Press back up to the starting position without letting your shoulders rise up the ears.

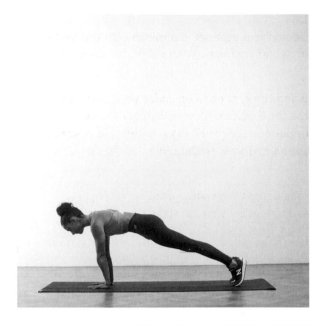

Key alignment cues
The elbows should shave the sides of your body as you rise up and drop into the push-up. Do not let your upper shoulders take over the movement; try to keep them relaxed. Avoid letting the body sag at the hips.

Main muscles worked
Triceps. The close grip push-up is a favourite variation for me because of the loading it puts on the triceps. Most women don't want large pectorals so this is the variation I emphasise for my female clients. Men also tend to neglect their tricep development and work on growing a massive chest and biceps (there is nothing wrong with that, but ladies love triceps too).

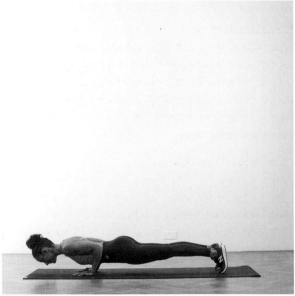

A3 BENT ARM REVERSE KETTLEBELL LUNGE

1.
Begin from a standing position with the kettlebell in the left hand, with your right hand on your hip.

2.
Bring the kettlebell up under your chin, with the 'bell' resting on your outer forearm and upper arm. Lift the elbow so that the weight is supported by your deltoid.

3.
Take a giant step back with the left leg, into a long lunge until your right leg comes into a 90-degree angle.

4.
Press through the right heel to stand up and drive your left knee up and forwards. Reverse these instructions for the left side.

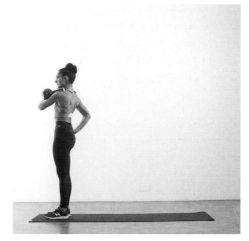

Key alignment cues
Keep the spine neutral at all times and avoid letting your lower belly relax. Keep it lightly pulled inwards. To really activate your glute in this movement, ensure that your ankle does not go beyond the toes. Press through the heel to stand up out of the lunge.

Main muscles worked
This is a knee-dominant movement, so technically speaking it really works your quads. However, I tweak all my lunges by making them extra-long in stance so that my hamstrings and glutes have to fire to get me out of the deep lunge.

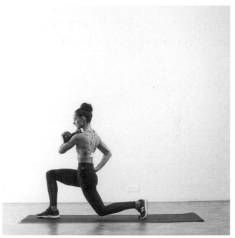

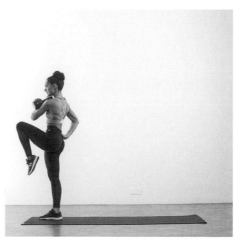

A4 LUNGE STANCE SINGLE ARM ROW

1.
Step into a long lunge with the right leg leading and bend forward from the hips.

2.
Using the left hand, pick up the kettlebell and hold it, while keeping your lower back straight and belly button hugging towards the spine. This is the starting position.

3.
Exhale and pull the kettlebell straight up to the side of your chest, keeping your upper arm close to your side and keeping the body still (no movement through the torso).

4.
Inhale and return to the starting position.

5.
Repeat as directed, then switch sides.

Key alignment cues
The spine must stay neutral; do not let your upper back round. You want to lead the movement from your shoulder blade rather than your arm. Drive the front heel into the ground for extra isometric contractions of the glutes.

Main muscles worked
Middle back, lower trapezius, some latissimus dorsi as well as deep anti-rotational core muscles. Your glutes will feel sore after this too.

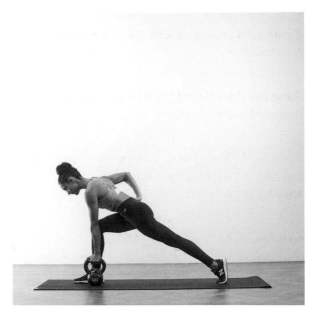

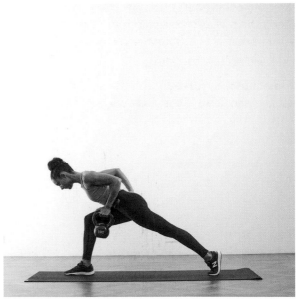

B1 KETTLEBELL SINGLE LEG GLUTE BRIDGE

1.
Come onto your back with your knees bent and feet together.

2.
Raise the right leg off the floor, bending the knee in towards your chest.

3.
Place the kettlebell over your left hip and push the right heel into the floor, driving your hips up towards the ceiling.

4.
Return to the starting position.

5.
Repeat as directed, then switch sides.

Key alignment cues
Keep the raised knee close towards your chest to ensure that your tailbone remains tucked. Keep your shoulders relaxed.

Main muscles worked
Glutes and hamstrings – all the good stuff.

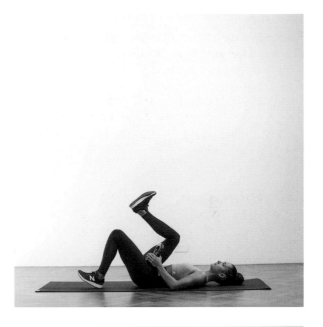

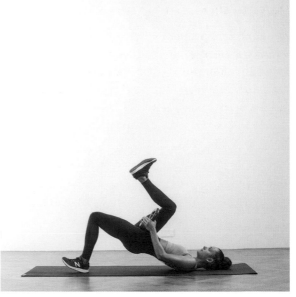

B2 SIDE LYING HIP RAISE

1.
Roll over onto your right side, placing your right elbow underneath your right shoulder. Ensure your palm is down and the forearm and wrist are in line with the elbow. Bend your right leg at a 45-degree angle. Ensure that your hip and ankle are in alignment. Straighten the left leg and lift the left ankle off the floor. This is your starting position.

2.
Push into the right knee (with some support from the elbow), lifting your hips off the floor.

3.
Lower back down to the starting position for repetition.

4.
Repeat as directed, then switch sides.

Key alignment cues
Keep your core tight; imagine wearing a corset. There should be no movement between the ribs and hips.

Main muscles worked
This is such a glute burner, and of course your shoulder will feel a little worked as well. If you feel it in your back, it usually means that your erectors and quadratus lumborom (back muscles) are trying to do the work, rather than the glutes.

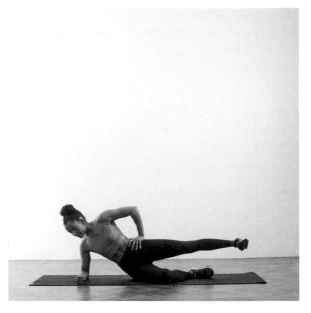

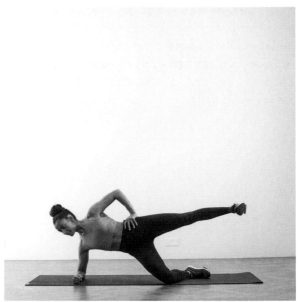

C1 REVERSE CRUNCH

1.
Lie on your back, placing your heavy kettlebell about 15cm from your head and hold onto the 'bell' section.

2.
Draw the belly button to the spine and, using the engagement of your abdominals, lift your hips high.

3.
Lower the spine back to the floor, one vertebra at a time.

Key alignment cues
It's really important that you feel the sensation of curling the spine back down to the ground, otherwise you may feel this exercise more in the lower back rather than the abdominals.

Main muscles worked
If performed correctly this exercise really helps to recruit the lower abs, as well as the upper rectus abdominus.

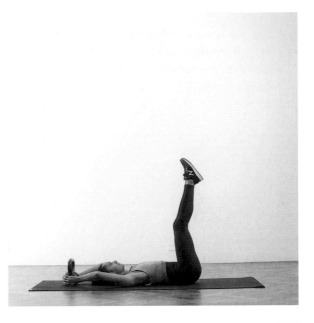

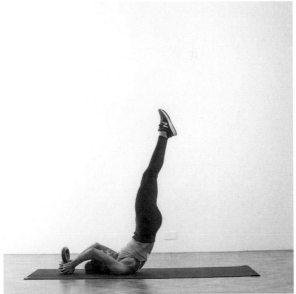

C2 KETTLEBELL CRUNCH

1.
Grab your kettlebell and bring it onto your chest. Come onto your back with your knees bent and feet hip distance apart, raising the toes off the floor.

2.
Straighten your arms up towards the ceiling, keeping your neck long and shoulders relaxed.

3.
Begin to curl the spine off the floor, until your middle back only lifts off, pressing the kettlebell up towards the ceiling.

4.
Lower back down with control, rolling down one vertebra at a time to the floor.

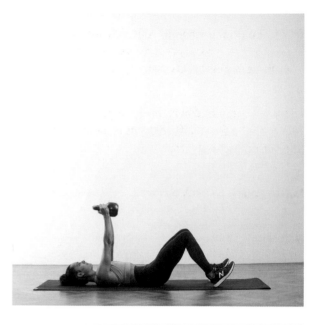

Key alignment cues
Draw the lower belly in before you move. Keep the neck and shoulders as relaxed as possible. Use your abs.

Main muscles worked
Rectus abdominus (six-pack) as well as the deeper core.

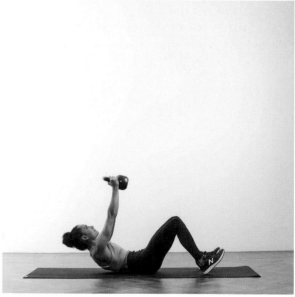

C3 TABLE TOP ROCKS

1.
Sit on the floor with your feet in front of you, knees bent and hands resting behind you with your fingers pointing towards you.

2.
Lift your chest and hips, pushing your hands and feet into the floor. Lift the hips until they are in line with the shoulders.

3.
Lower your hips back down to the floor.

Key alignment cues
Draw your belly in the whole time, and tuck your tail bone at the top of the movement. Don't forget to lift through the chest. Keep your head in line with the rest of the spine.

Main muscles worked
This is an awesome shoulder and bicep mobility drill, but also works the posterior muscles too, like hamstrings and glutes.

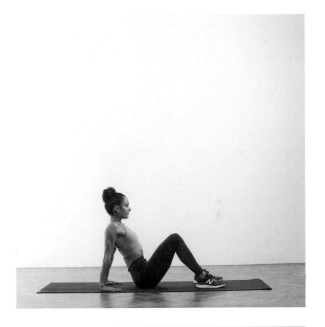

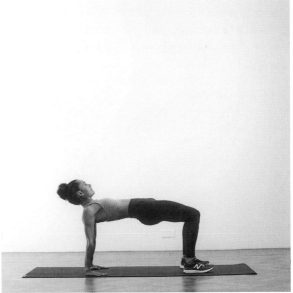

C4 PUSH-UP TO BIRD DOG

1.
Come into a push-up position and lower down,
an inch off the floor.

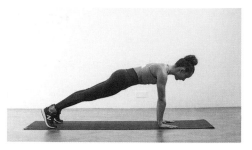

2.
Push back up to the top push-up position and lift
the left arm and right leg off the floor, balancing.

3.
Return to the push-up position and repeat as
directed, alternating sides.

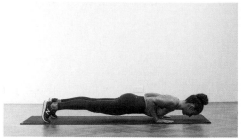

Key alignment cues
Do not let your body sag at any point of this
movement, especially during the Bird Dog
section. Ensure that your abs are tight for the
entire set and keep this one fast and dynamic.

Main muscles worked
This is actually a full-body activating exercise,
however it also works to train contralateral
stability (stability between the left and right sides
of you). The plank position works your anterior
muscles and the Bird Dog variation works your
posterior muscles.

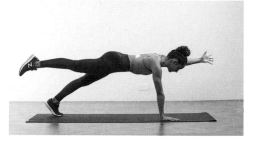

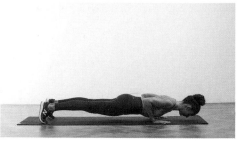

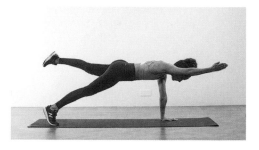

ADVANCED – VM WORKOUT 2

	EXERCISE	REPS	TEMPO	REST
A1 L & R	Shoulder Elevated Single Leg Hip Thrust (page 174)	12–15	2110	10s
A2	Wide Grip Push-up (page 175)	10–12	3010	10s
A3 L & R	KB Split Squat (Back Foot Raise) (page 176)	12–15	2010	10s
A4	Kettlebell Pullover in Deadbug Position (page 177)	10–12	2010	30s
	REPEAT X 3 SETS			
B1 L & R	Kettlebell Single Leg Squat (page 178)	12–15	1010	10s
B2 L & R	Banded Kickback (page 179)	12–15	1010	30s
	REPEAT X 3 SETS			
C1	Alternating Step Up with Kettlebell (page 180)	15	1010	10s
C2	Seated Band Abduction (page 181)	15	1010	10s
	REPEAT X 2 SETS			
D1 L & R	Kettlebell Standing Side Bend (page 182)	15	1010	10s
D2 L & R	Side Plank Hip Raise (page 183)	15	1010	20s
	REPEAT X 3 SETS			
E1	Bicycles (page 184)	30	1010	30s
	REPEAT X 3 SETS			

IF YOU'RE GOING TO THE GYM DON'T FORGET TO TAKE A PHOTO OF THIS PAGE WITH YOUR PHONE SO YOU CAN DO THE WORKOUT.

A1 SHOULDER ELEVATED SINGLE LEG HIP THRUST

1.
Begin by sitting with the backs of your shoulders up against your chair/bench, placing the kettlebell on your right hip.

2.
Pushing through your heels, lift your hips towards the ceiling until they align with the height of your shoulders. Squeeze your glutes. Lift the left leg. This is your starting position.

3.
Keeping your left leg in the air, lower your hips towards the floor without them touching the ground.

4.
Shoot your hips back up (only using that right leg, as the left leg is in the air).

5.
Repeat as directed, then switch sides.

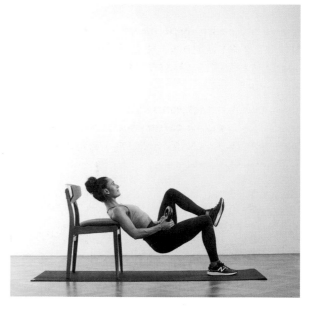

Key alignment cues
Dig the supporting heel into the floor, draw your tummy in and tuck your tail bone as though you wanted to push your pubic bone towards the ceiling. Watch out for bending of the lower back; try to lengthen out the lower spine.

Main muscles worked
Glutes, baby, this should be all about the glutes. Some hamstring and very minimal quads.

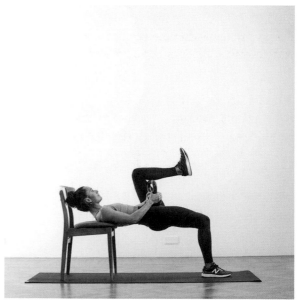

A2 WIDE GRIP PUSH-UP

1.
Come into a push-up position with the hands just over shoulder distance apart. Make sure your wrists are stacked just under the shoulders.

2.
Walk your feet backwards so that your hips can extend, allowing for correct spinal and pelvic alignment. You should be in one long line from head to feet.

3.
Take a deep breath in, bend at the elbows and begin to lower the chest towards the floor. Keep the elbows close as you lower towards the floor.

4.
Go as deep as possible into the push-up while maintaining integrity to the spine and pelvis.

5.
Press back up to the starting position without letting your shoulders rise up the ears.

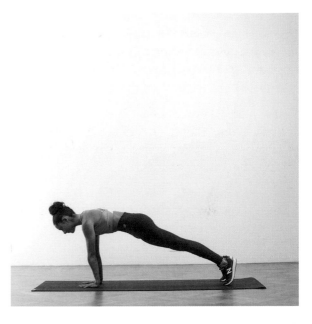

Key alignment cues
Avoid letting your hips sag towards the floor. Keep the neck long, and try to avoid letting the upper trapezius take over, keeping the shoulders away from the ears.

Main muscles worked
Pectorals.

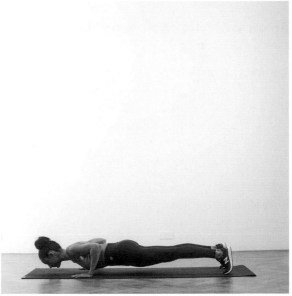

A3 KETTLEBELL SPLIT SQUAT (BACK FOOT RAISED)

1.
Take the kettlebell in your left hand, bring it up under your chin, with the 'bell' resting on your outer forearm and upper arm. Lift the elbow so that the weight is supported by your deltoid.

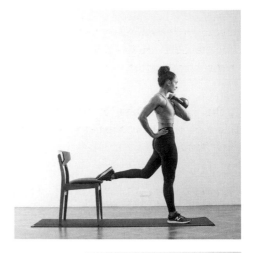

2.
Facing away from your chair/bench, shift your body weight onto the right leg and lift the left leg up onto the chair/bench behind you. Place your foot on the chair with your shoelaces facing down. Hop your front leg a little further forward so you are in a fairly long stance.

3.
Bend both knees and begin to lower the back knee towards the floor. Let the kettlebell touch the floor.

4.
Return to the top of the lunge quickly.

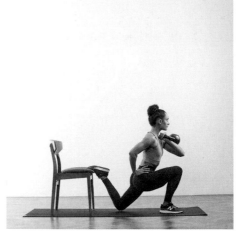

5.
Repeat as directed, then switch sides.

Key alignment cues
Avoid overarching the lower back when you get to the bottom of the lunge. If you feel tight in the quad of the raised leg, bend the knee more. Keep the weight in the heel of the front foot. A slight lean forward will help you to feel this a little more in the glutes.

Main muscles worked
Glutes and hamstrings. It's also great for increasing flexibility.

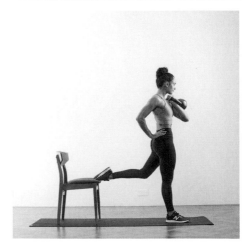

A4 KETTLEBELL PULLOVER IN DEADBUG POSITION

1.
Holding your kettlebell by the horns, come onto your back in a table-top position with your arms straight above your chest.

2.
Keeping the ribs in and belly button drawn towards the spine, begin to extend the kettlebell above your head.

3.
Bring the kettlebell back to the starting position and repeat.

Key alignment cues
Avoid letting your lower back come off the floor, keep your ribs flat and your neck relaxed.

Main muscles worked
The lats and abs.

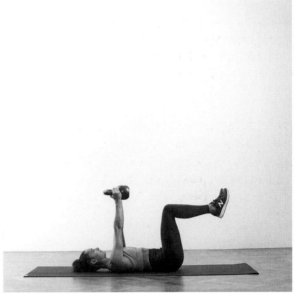

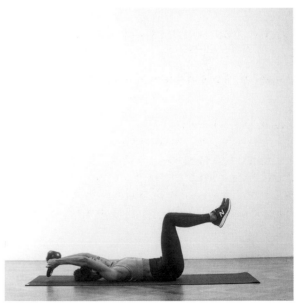

B1 KETTLEBELL SINGLE LEG SQUAT (to the chair or bench)

1.
Grab your kettlebell and bring it up under the chin. The bell will be resting on your outer forearm and upper arm.

2.
Stand facing away from the chair/bench. Placing your hands on your hips, raise the left leg.

3.
Keeping your chest tall, push your hips back and start to squat towards the chair behind you.

4.
Sit all the way down, then drive up back to the standing position. Do not let your raised leg touch the floor.

5.
Repeat as directed, then switch sides.

Key alignment cues
It will be really tempting to let your supporting heel come off the floor as you lower into the squat. Push the hips backwards and try to imitate the same stature that you would have in a regular squat.

Main muscles worked
Glutes and quads.

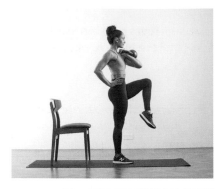

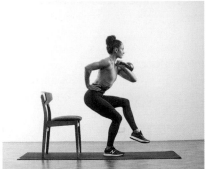

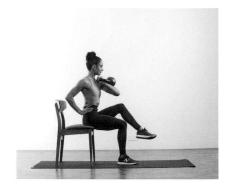

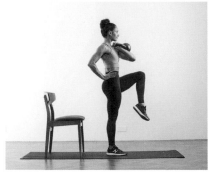

B2 BANDED KICKBACK

1.
Come into an all-fours position inside of the band, with one edge of the band hooked around the thumbs.

2.
Hook the other side of the band around your right heel and extend the right leg, squeezing the glute against the resistance.

3.
Return to centre and repeat as directed, then switch sides.

Key alignment cues
Avoid letting the hips lift or tilt and maintain a neutral spine. You will want to bend the lower back as you extend your leg, but it's important to use your core and shoulder stability to stop this from happening, to fully work your glutes.

Main muscles worked
Glutes and quads.

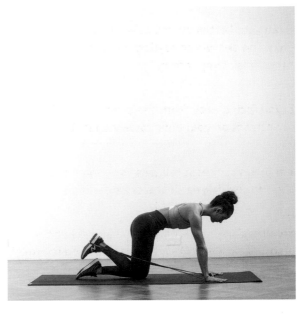

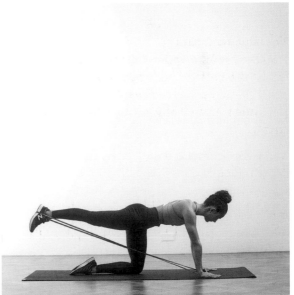

C1 ALTERNATING STEP UP WITH KETTLEBELL

1.
Facing your chair/bench, place the right foot on top of it while holding the kettlebell in your left hand. Place your right hand on your hip and lift through the chest.

2.
Drive through the heel of your right leg (trying your best not to push off the left) and step up onto the chair.

3.
Step your left foot back down to the ground.

4.
Swap the kettlebell to the right hand.

5.
Drive through the heel of your left leg (trying your best not to push off the right) and step up onto the chair.

6.
Repeat this movement dynamically, alternating sides, making sure that you swap the kettlebell.

Key alignment cues
Make this more about your glutes, by leaning forwards slightly (to create a stretch in the hamstrings and glutes) and drive through the heel to stand up.

Main muscles worked
Glutes and quads.

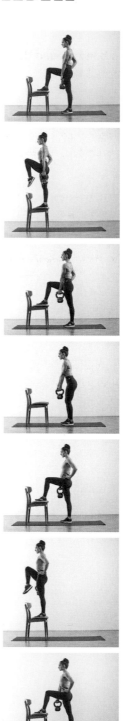

C2 SEATED BAND ABDUCTION

1.
Place the looped band around the knees (remember to loop it twice).

2.
Sit on the edge of your chair/bench, with your hands on your hips, chest lifted. Lean forward slightly, pushing your hips back.

3.
Push the knees out wide against the band as far as you can.

4.
Return to the starting position, then repeat.

Key alignment cues
Avoid rounding your lower back. Keep the chest lifted and the shoulders relaxed.

Main muscles worked
Gluteals (particularly gluteus medius).

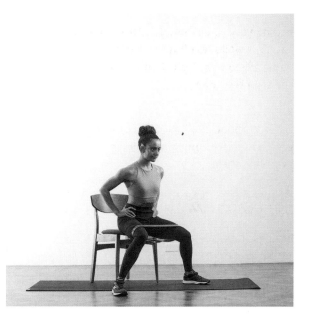

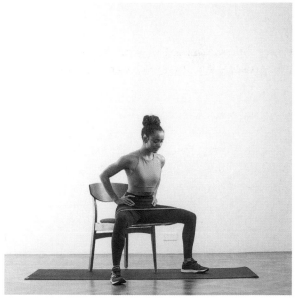

D1 KETTLEBELL STANDING SIDE BEND

1.
Stand upright with your kettlebell in your left hand, by your side and your right hand resting on the back of your head.

2.
Bend sideways to the left until your kettlebell touches just below your knee, and then straighten to the original position.

3.
Repeat as directed, then switch sides.

Key alignment cues
It's extremely important to keep your chest lifted and spine long during this entire motion. Think about bending sideways, while keeping your hips still.

Main muscles worked
Obliques.

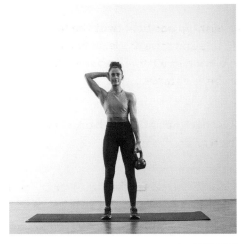

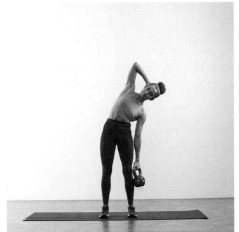

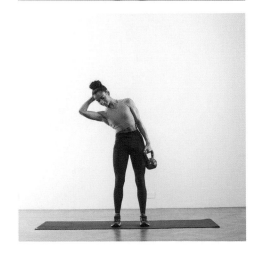

D2 SIDE PLANK HIP RAISE

1.
From a push-up position, twist the heels to the left side and raise the left hand off the floor. It should bring you into a high side plank position. This will be the starting pose.

2.
Take your right hand to your hip and lower the hips down to the floor.

3.
Using your obliques, lift the hips back up as high as you possibly can.

4.
Repeat as directed, then switch sides.

Key alignment cues
If you feel this in your lower back, tip the top hip down slightly. Make sure your head stays in alignment with your body.

Main muscles worked
Obliques and shoulders.

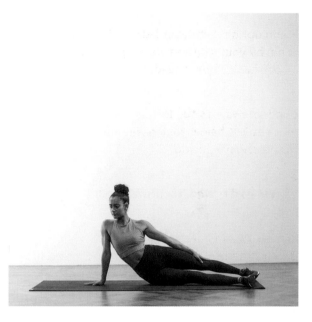

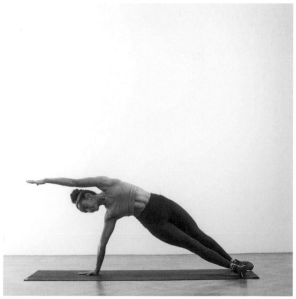

E1 BICYCLES

1.
Lie on your back with the knees bent up towards the ceiling.

2.
Place your fingers onto your ears, flex and rotate the upper spine by raising the upper body off the ground. Your shoulder blades should not be on the floor.

3.
Twist to bring the elbow to its opposing knee and vice versa.

4.
Repeat as directed, alternating sides.

Key alignment cues
Keep your belly button pulled inwardly towards the spine throughout the movement. Try not to let your lower back come off the floor.

Main muscles worked
Rectus abdominus (six-pack) and a little of the internal and external obliques.

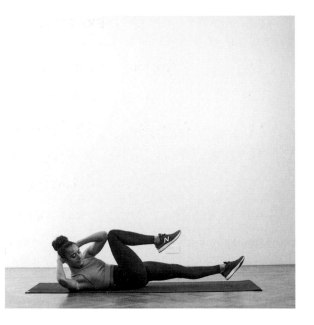

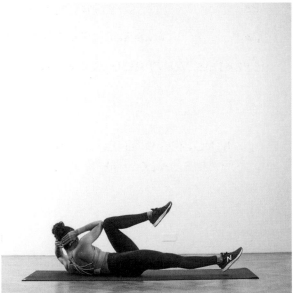

The Workouts

ADVANCED – VM WORKOUT 3 (CARDIO)

	EXERCISE	REPS	REST
A1	Alternating Plyometric Lunge (page 186)	20	0s
A2	Mountain Climbers (page 187)	20	0s
A3	Alternating Squat to Side Kick (page 188)	20	0s
A4	Full Burpees (page 189)	20	0s
A5	Sumo Squat Jump (page 190)	20	0s
A6	Shoulder Taps (page 191)	20	0s

REPEAT AS MANY ROUNDS AS POSSIBLE FOR 10 MINUTES

	EXERCISE	REPS	REST
B1	Hollow Body Hold (page 192)	45s	15s
B2	Russian Twist (page 193)	45s	15s
B3	V-ups (page 194)	45s	15s
B4	Towel Sliding Floor Pike (page 195)	45s	15s

REPEAT AS MANY ROUNDS AS POSSIBLE FOR 10 MINUTES

IF YOU'RE GOING TO THE GYM DON'T FORGET TO TAKE A PHOTO OF THIS PAGE WITH YOUR PHONE SO YOU CAN DO THE WORKOUT.

A1 ALTERNATING PLYOMETRIC LUNGE

1.
Begin from a standing position, placing your hands on your hips.

2.
Take a giant step back with the left leg into a long lunge, until your right leg comes into a 90-degree angle. This is the starting position.

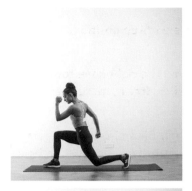

3.
Drive through the right heel and left foot to dynamically jump out of the lunge. Swap the legs in the air, landing onto the opposite side lunge with the left leg in front and right leg behind.

4.
Repeat as directed, alternating sides.

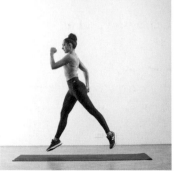

Key alignment cues
Plyometric movements are advanced because they require stability. If you don't yet feel very strong and stable in a dynamic alternating lunge, you should not be doing this variation.

Main muscles worked
This is a plyometric movement (explosive movement) that can be extremely effective and intense. It will really work your hamstrings and inner thighs if you go deep enough.

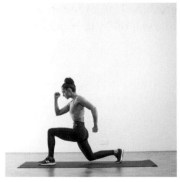

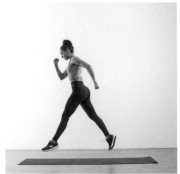

A2 MOUNTAIN CLIMBERS

1.
Move into a push-up position.

2.
Quickly bring the right knee towards the back of the right elbow (try to make them touch).

3.
In a fast, almost jumping motion, switch legs and try to touch the back of the left elbow with your left knee.

4.
Repeat as quickly as possible.

Key alignment cues
Suck your belly in during the entire movement. Keep it fast and dynamic and keep your hips at a neutral height, not higher or lower than the shoulders.

Main muscles worked
All-out everything kind of move, but if performed correctly, you will feel this in your lower abs too.

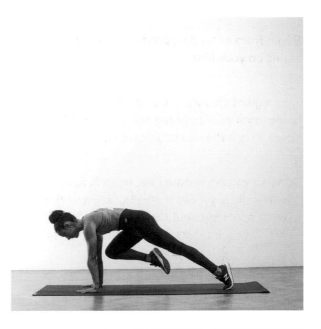

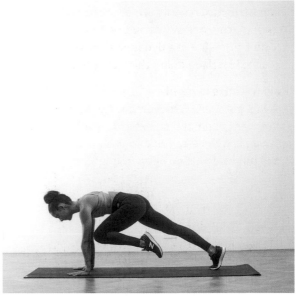

A3 ALTERNATING SQUAT TO SIDE KICK

1.
Take a squat stance (as instructed on page 126 but without the band) and move into your squat position.

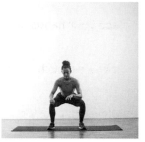

2.
As you begin to rise up and out of the squat, lean onto the left leg and side kick your right leg.

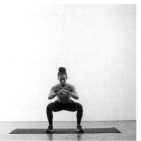

3.
Return back to the squat and prepare to kick to the left.

4.
Repeat this sequence, alternating sides.

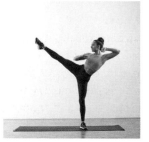

Key alignment cues
This is dynamic, but ensure that you still exercise the same neutral spine as in a usual squat. Just because it's fast, doesn't mean it should lose all focus.

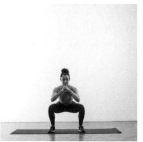

Main muscles worked
Glutes and hamstrings. It's also great for lifting the heart rate and adding some fire to the HIIT session.

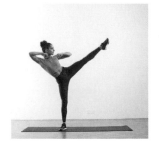

A4 FULL BURPEE

1.
Bend over and place your hands on the floor.

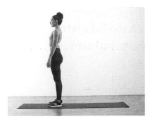

2.
Jump the feet back into a push-up position.

3.
Lower your body down to the floor.

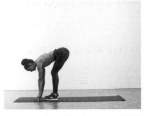

4.
Press back up to push-up position.

5.
Jump the feet back to the outsides of your hands.

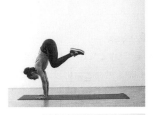

6.
Lift the body and jump up, reaching the arms upwards as you do.

Key alignment cues
Burpees are a great exercise aerobically, but realistically they aren't teaching you anything amazing about form or correct movement patterns. As best as possible, try to maintain all the cues for push-ups and squats that I've outlined in this book so that you are staying safe throughout this movement.

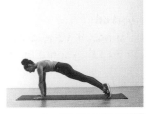

Main muscles worked
Everything. Especially the heart.

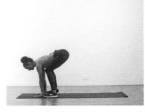

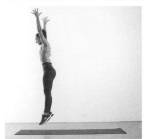

A5 SUMO SQUAT JUMP

1.
Take your feet much wider than shoulder distance apart and bring your palms together in front of your chest.

2.
Keeping your chest lifted, drop the hips down into a squat, keeping the spine neutral.

3.
Pushing into the heels, jump up out of the squat. Land softly, bending the knees.

4.
Repeat as directed.

Key alignment cues
Maintain those squatting principles I have outlined already, but try to move quickly and dynamically. Keep your chest up at all times and do not let the spine round.

Main muscles worked
Glutes, hamstrings and adductors.

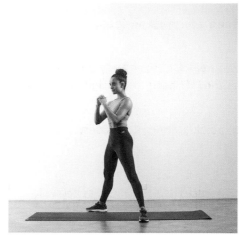

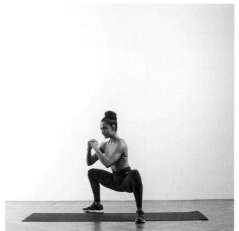

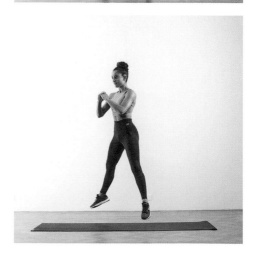

A6 SHOULDER TAPS

1.
Come into a push-up position.

2.
Shift the weight of your body onto the right side
and tap the left hand to the right shoulder.

3.
Repeat quickly, alternating sides.

Key alignment cues
Use your anti-rotational muscles to avoid letting
the hips move from side to side. Do NOT let your
hips sag towards the floor.

Main muscles worked
Core stabilisers.

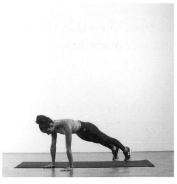

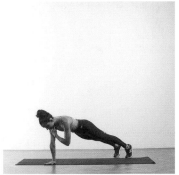

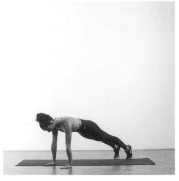

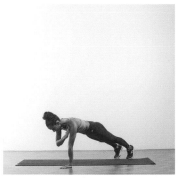

B1 HOLLOW BODY HOLD

1.
Lying on your back, draw the belly button down towards the floor, and press your lower spine into the floor.

2.
Keep your abs and butt tight at all times, extend your arms above your head and curl your upper spine and shoulders off the floor.

3.
Slowly raise the legs off the floor, making a dish shape with your body.

4.
Hold here for the time specified.

Key alignment cues
Try to maintain a dish-like position without losing integrity of the spine. Belly stays flat.

Main muscles worked
Abdominals.

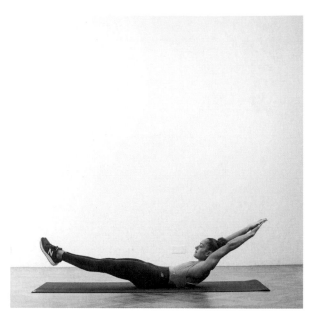

B2 RUSSIAN TWIST

1.
Come into a seated position with your legs extended out in front of you, and knees slightly bent.

2.
With your arms close to your body, bring one hand onto the other with your elbows bent, lean back and gently lift your legs off the floor so that you are balancing on your buttocks. This is the starting position.

3.
Twisting from the torso, move your shoulders, arms and hands around to the left.

4.
Return to the centre and repeat on the right side.

5.
Repeat as directed, continuing to alternate sides for the time specified.

Key alignment cues
Draw the belly button in toward the spine, while keeping the lower spine as neutral as possible. Avoid excessive arching of the lower back, this may be an indicator that you're using your hip flexors more than your abdominals.

Main muscles worked
Because this is a twisting abdominal exercise there is emphasis on the obliques, however if performed correctly it will hit all of your abdominal muscles.

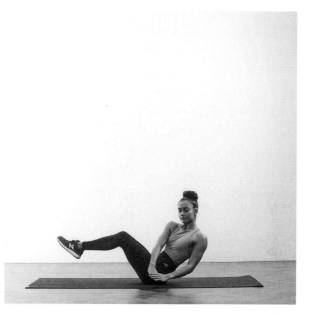

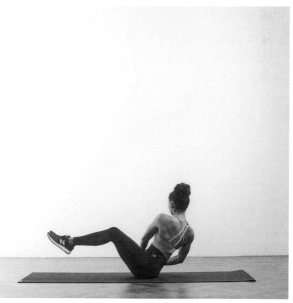

B3 V-UPS

1.
Lie on your back with your arms and legs extended straight. This will be your starting position.

2.
As you exhale, bend at the waist and raise your legs and arms to meet in a V position.

3.
While inhaling, lower your arms and legs back to the starting position.

4.
Repeat.

Key alignment cues
If this feels too difficult, let your knees bend so that it becomes a tuck-up. As you come back into the extended position, ensure your belly button is drawing in towards the spine, your tummy is flat and your core is tight.

Main muscles worked
Rectus abdominus (six-pack) and a little of the internal and external obliques.

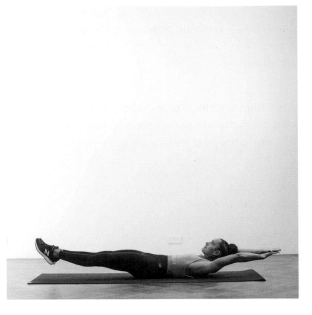

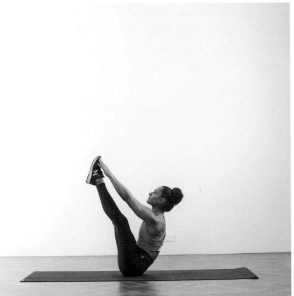

B4 TOWEL SLIDING FLOOR PIKE

1.
Come into a push-up position with your feet placed on a towel, keeping your toes straight not tucked.

2.
Lean the shoulders forward, press your palms into the floor and slide your body into a piked position with your hips in the air.

3.
Return to the starting position and repeat for the specified time.

Key alignment cues
Feel the sensation of sucking the belly in throughout the entire exercise. Avoid letting your hips sag to the floor in the push-up position.

Main muscles worked
Shoulders and whole core. You will feel almost every muscle in your body working in this exercise.

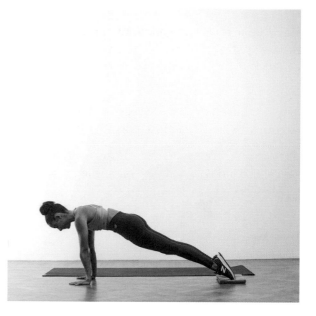

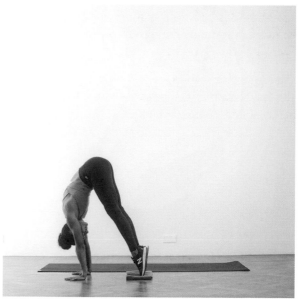

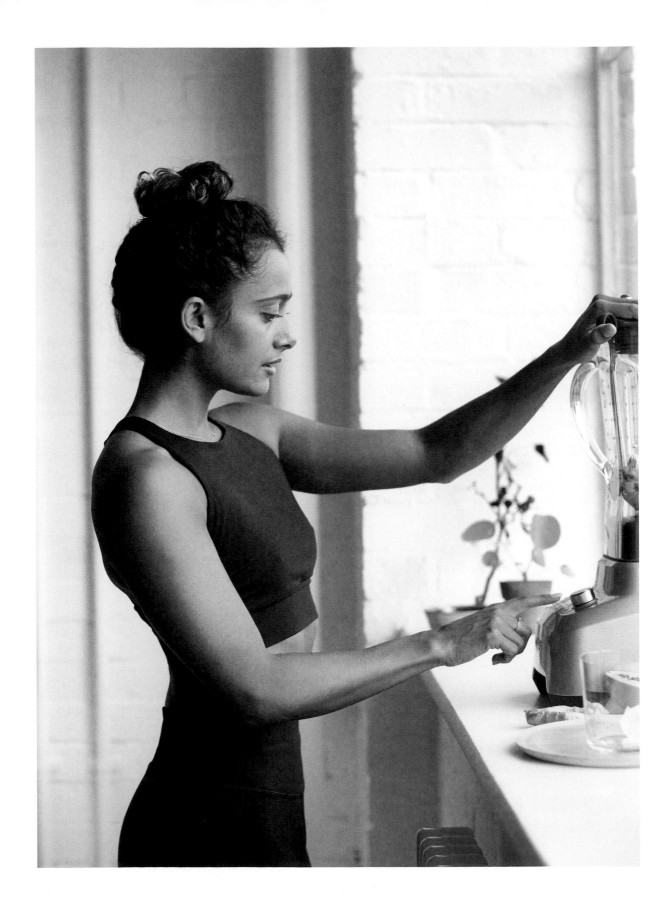

THE FOOD PLAN

Food plans have the potential to reinforce dangerous (often subconscious) tendencies of labelling foods as 'good' or 'bad', and I don't want you thinking that if a particular food ingredient is not on my food plan, that it is 'evil'. That being said, the 28-day reset plan is designed to help you do exactly that – reset. Months of drinking alcohol a few nights a week, regularly eating processed foods to save time or frequently bingeing on ice cream can cause us to disconnect a little from how food affects our body.

My 28-day reset plan is not a depressingly low-calorie, low-carb diet (phew). In fact, it's going to be bespoke, because you are going to add your protein content into the various vegetable meals, while following a few cooking rules as well. I know that some of you are meat eaters and others are vegans – so all you have to do is measure up your protein sources so that you are hitting your required protein targets then pick a favourite salad or veggie dish to accompany it.

There's no denying that eating vegetables is good for us. They are packed with an abundance of micronutrients and it's really important that we get them into our diets. In fact, in my food plan, the salads and vegetable dishes are the star of the show. That way I know you will be always getting a sufficient amount.

On each of the 28 days you will consume one of each of these meals:

Breakfast (there are seven to choose from –try to mix them as often as possible as consuming different breakfasts will provide you with a range of micronutrients)

Vertueous Veggie Box (with your added palm-sized portion of protein – or two palm-sized portions for vegans)

Dinner (either a Booty-full Bowl on weights days or Lean Greens on cardio days, with your added protein)

Smoothie (you can have this for dessert or any time throughout the day. I prefer to have these as my sweet treat after dinner or at that 4pm munchies craving time)

Breakfast and Smoothie recipes contain around 20–24g protein already. Lunch and Dinner meals usually require your protein portion (vegans will require two portions).

THE SET UP

'Fail to prepare, prepare to fail.' I know that statement sounds a little harsh, and I don't really like the word fail, but if you lead a busy life, then it will really apply to you. Get ready to prep for the next 28 days so that you find an easy routine. If you feel ill-equipped, you'll find reasons to skip meals or eat something else on the go. I'm not expecting you to prep your meals and fill your kitchen with 100 Tupperware boxes (which is also bad for the environment). I simply want you to prepare your kitchen and have a good understanding of some simple techniques before you begin.

Cooking Vertueously

Cooking your vegetables – I prefer to steam my vegetables to help retain the nutrient content. When you boil vegetables you often lose the nutrient content into the water. This would be okay in the case of soup, but if you're not going to consume the 'vegetable water', you'll be losing out on valuable vitamins and minerals.

Cooking your meat and poultry –There are lots of great ways to cook meat in a healthy way. Pan- or wok-fried meat, cooked in coconut oil, butter or olive oil, is a great and convenient option. Here's a quick method for getting flavoursome meat:
— Slice up your palm-sized portion of meat and season with salt and pepper.
— Pan-fry the meat on a medium to high heat in 1 tsp coconut oil, olive oil or butter, for 2–3 minutes (for chicken) or 3–4 minutes (for red meat), or until cooked to your liking.
— Add in ½ tsp chopped garlic and 1 tsp finely chopped ginger, cooking for a further minute. Be creative with your herbs and spices: oregano, thyme, rosemary, sage, turmeric and Chinese five-spice are all great ways to flavour meat. Do make sure you throw them in before the meat is cooked, though, so that the meat absorbs the flavours.

Cooking your fish – I personally find the easiest (and least smelly) way to cook fish is to oven bake it, but if you find it easier to pan-fry, go ahead.
— Preheat the oven to 180°C/gas 4.
— Take your palm-sized portion of fish and place it on a piece of baking parchment that's large enough to fit around the fish and be able to wrap it loosely.
— Mix 1 tsp extra virgin olive oil, 1 tsp light soy sauce, 1 tsp finely chopped ginger and a dollop of honey in a small bowl, to make a marinade.
— Drizzle the marinade over the fish and fold up the edges of the paper to form

a 'bag' around the fish. Fold or twist the edges to seal the bag.
— Place on a baking tray and bake in the oven for 20–30 minutes, depending
  on the thickness of your fish.
— Play around with marinade options. Lemon juice, sea salt and olive oil is another
  simple and delicious summer option.

Cooking your vegetarian protein – I love eggs. They are my go-to source of protein
most of the time and I will very often cook up some extra boiled eggs to drop into
my salads, or cook an extra egg-white omelette, so that I am not overdoing my fat
allowance for the day. Remember that 1 large egg has roughly 6g protein so you
will need around 3–4 eggs to get a 20–24g serving. This is why I will often use egg
whites, as 4 eggs also contain 20g total fat, making it hard to stick to my RDI of fat.
This omelette recipe is easy and you just need to throw it on top of any of my meals:
— Melt ½ tsp coconut oil or butter in a pan.
— Pour 175ml egg whites into the pan and allow to cook.
— Sprinkle your favourite herbs over the omelette as it cooks.
— Once the base has set, fold the omelette in half, remove from the heat and leave
  in the pan for 2 minutes, to cook further.

Cooking your vegan protein –If the protein you're using is vegan you're going to need
roughly two palm-sized servings, and to ensure you're getting lots of different amino
acids try two different types. An example would be, one serving of tofu and another
of boiled black beans. My favourite way to cook tofu is to pan-fry it:
— Take your tofu out of the packet, place it between 2 sheets of kitchen paper
  and place something heavy on top of it. Leave for 10–20 minutes to press the
  extra liquid out (trust me, this is the key to making delicious and crispy tofu).
— Slice it to your desired thickness and shape.
— Heat 1 tsp olive oil in a pan with 1 tsp chopped garlic and 2 tsp sliced ginger.
  Add the tofu to the pan.
— The tofu slices need to be browned on one side before you flip them – allow to
  cook until it frees from the pan, then cook the other side.

If you're using pre-cooked grains and legumes, ensure that you follow the packet
instructions to warm them up. I heat mine in a pan with some light seasoning.
For lentils I will add some turmeric, paprika and pepper (with ½ tsp coconut oil
and 1 tbsp water). For kidney beans I like to use a Mexican spice mix.

PIMP YOUR PROTEIN

In the words of the Spice Girls, I really believe it's important to 'spice up your life' – or in this case, spice up your protein. If your food has no taste, you're going to lose inspiration. The last thing I want is for you to lose interest in your food because you feel that it lacks flavour and intensity. Rather than you reaching for that highly processed and sugar-loaded bottle of red sauce to flavour up your protein, I have listed below some of my absolute favourite marinades.

Simply mix up the ingredients and then gently massage into your protein servings. Obviously, the longer you leave it in the marinade the better, and placing it in a lunchbox in the fridge overnight can be a great way to let the flavours absorb. However, if you're anything like me, you don't and can't think that far ahead, so just setting it aside for a few minutes is another option.

Five spice marinade
1 tbsp light soy sauce
1 tsp Chinese five-spice powder
1 tsp honey
1 tsp crushed garlic
1 tbsp olive oil

Lemon, garlic and herb marinade
juice of ½ lemon
1 tsp finely chopped garlic
1 tbsp olive oil
1 tsp thyme leaves
a pinch of sea salt

Honey balsamic marinade
1 tsp honey
1 tsp balsamic vinegar
1 tsp olive oil
½ tsp finely chopped garlic
1 tsp sesame seeds
(optional; sprinkle over at the end of cooking)

Lime, honey, garlic and coriander marinade
juice of ½ lime
1 tsp honey
1 garlic clove, crushed
1 tbsp chopped coriander
1 tsp olive oil

Ginger, garlic and chilli marinade
1 tsp finely chopped ginger
1 tsp finely chopped garlic
a pinch of chilli flakes
1 tbsp olive oil

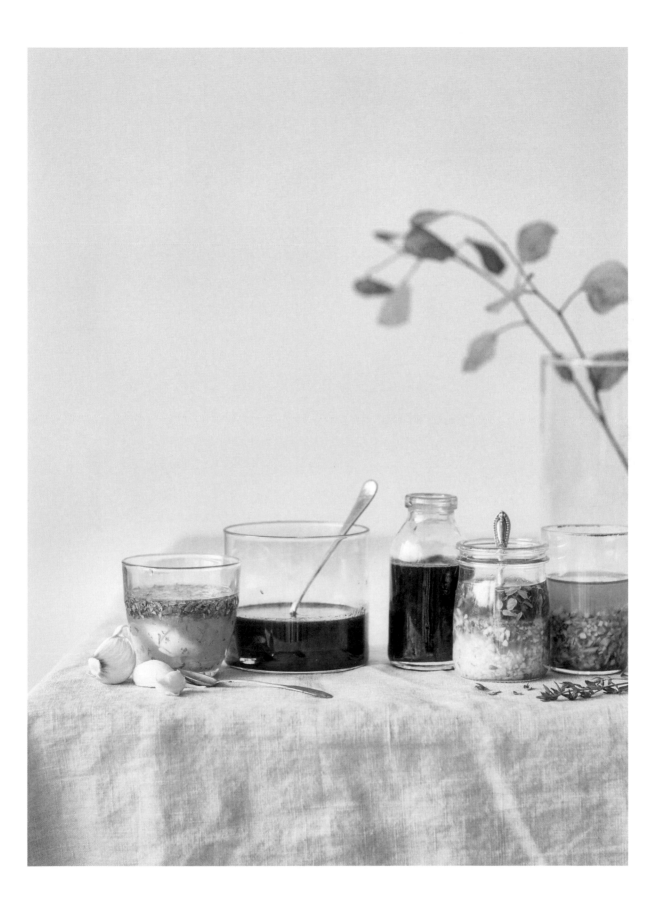

BREAKFAST

This is by far my favourite meal of the day, particularly because I wake up very hungry from that long, overnight fast. To me, eating when you're hungry feels right and good and delicious!

Even though breakfast was once promoted as being the most important meal of the day, the research suggests that it is no more metabolically important than lunch or dinner. Some studies have shown that a higher protein, lower glycaemic load (lower carb) breakfast choice can lead to better energy levels, and I personally have found this to be true of my own body. Protein (or more specifically amino acids) are important in the production of dopamine, the neurotransmitter that plays a big part in motor control and makes you feel motivated. As you will know by now, I am big on protein (or at least amino acids) so all these breakfasts contain 20g or more of protein. This also means that there is no need to add any.

I am just as rushed as you probably are in the mornings so don't worry, the recipes are all super speedy and delicious.

All recipes serve one.

PROPER SCRAMBLED EGGS
WITH CHIVES AND CHERRY TOMATOES

For me, scrambled eggs should be buttery and flavoursome, and the best way to do this is to add butter, of course; I also like to add a little cream. This dish is simple and easy to make, so is ideal for the mornings – many people tell me that they prefer to eat oats because they are quick and easy, but this dish takes roughly the same amount of time to prepare.

1 tsp butter
2 large eggs and 1 egg white, lightly beaten
1 tsp cream
3 cherry tomatoes, halved
1 tbsp chopped chives
sea salt (optional)

Heat the butter in a pan until melted, then immediately add the eggs. Cook, stirring, and taking it on and off the heat every minute.

Once the eggs have almost reached your desired scramble consistency (some like it really runny; I like it really fluffy), throw in the cream, tomatoes and chives and continue to stir.

Remove from the heat and tip onto a plate.

Sprinkle with sea salt, if you like, and chow down.

WARM PROTEIN ZOATS

This dish is called zoats because it is a combination of zucchini and oats (in Australia and America courgettes are known by their Italian name zucchini).

I love zoats because they are a sneaky way to get your greens intake up without feeling like a rabbit munching on vegetables all day. It seems strange to put a vegetable into a sweet dish, but I promise you won't taste the courgette, this will just taste like a regular bowl of oats. The consistency of your zoats will vary slightly depending on the type of protein powder you choose. Those of you using whey protein will notice quite a liquid consistency and the quantity of milk I've listed will be fine; however, those of you opting for a vegan powder will find that the liquid is absorbed quickly, leaving the oats drier so you may need to add more liquid. I believe that the consistency of your oats is a preference that holds the same importance as how you like your tea. Play around with the amount of liquid to get yours exactly how you like them.

50g rolled oats
1 small courgette (zucchini), finely grated
150ml fortified unsweetened rice or oat milk (though see note above)
1 tsp chia seeds
20g scoop vanilla protein powder
1 medium banana, sliced
1 tsp ground cinnamon
1 tsp coconut flakes

Put the oats, courgette, rice or oat milk, chia seeds and protein powder into a pan and bring to the boil, stirring regularly.

Once boiling, take off the heat and let it sit for 5–7 minutes, stirring frequently.

Pour into a bowl, top with the sliced banana, cinnamon and coconut flakes and serve.

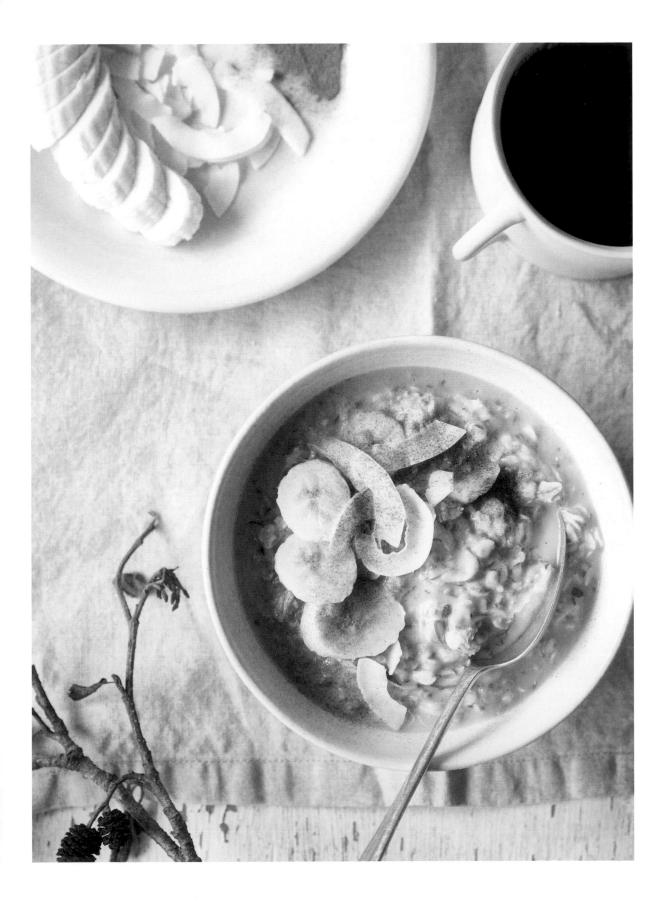

I-CAN'T-BELIEVE-IT'S-NOT-PIZZA OMELETTE

I am obsessed with pizza, in fact I actually think I should have been born Italian, as I consider myself to be something of a connoisseur. By no means is this recipe supposed to be a substitute for the delicious doughy delights of real Italian pizza. However, the flavours are almost identical and I promise that you will be pleasantly surprised by its similarities.

2 tsp olive oil
½ small onion, chopped
4 cherry tomatoes, chopped
3 mushrooms, chopped
a pinch of dried Italian herbs
2 large eggs and 1 egg white, lightly beaten
30g low-fat feta cheese
sea salt
a handful (about 20g) of watercress, to serve

Heat the olive oil in a frying pan, add the onion and cook until golden. Add the tomatoes, mushrooms and dried herbs and cook for 2 minutes.

Transfer the cooked vegetables to a plate or dish and return the pan to the heat.

Pour in the beaten eggs and allow to cook until just set, then add the cooked vegetables to one half of the omelette and crumble over the feta. Fold over the other side of the omelette, remove from the heat and leave in the pan for 2 minutes, to cook further.

Slide the omelette onto a plate, taking care, as you want to protect its Instagram-photo worthiness!

Sprinkle over some sea salt and serve with the watercress leaves.

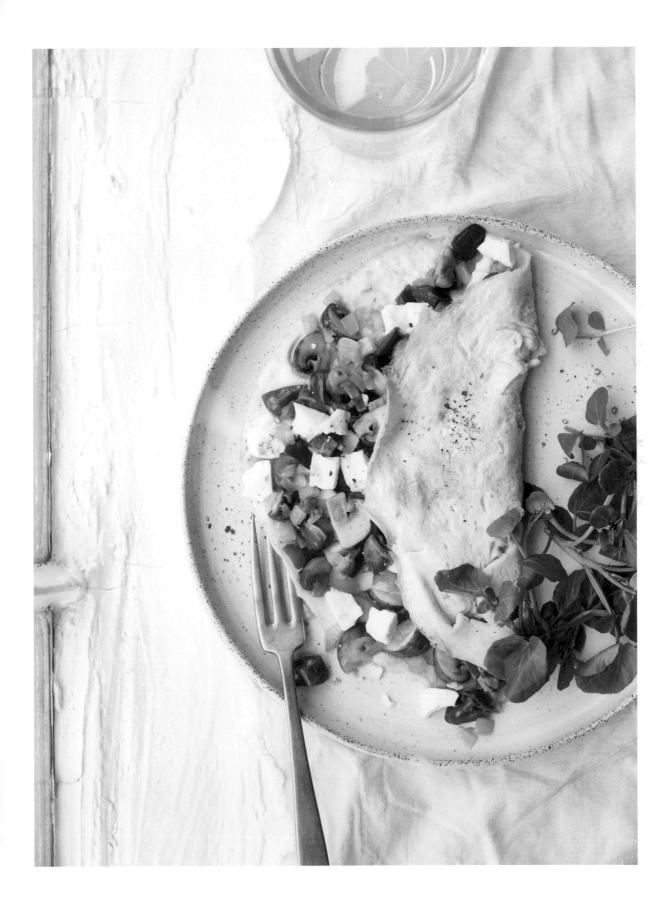

GREEN OMELETTE

I think that by now you are well aware of my obsession with vegetables, but the truth is I never used to like them very much. This recipe came about a while ago when I was trying to figure out ways to sneak more veg into my diet without my veggie-sceptic self noticing them. I know it's ridiculous, but for those of you who can relate to this, you will love this recipe. Quick, easy and packing a health punch in terms of its green nutrients, it's a staple for me at any time of the day.

2 tsp olive oil
½ tsp crushed garlic
½ courgette (zucchini), grated
a handful of baby spinach
1 tbsp chopped chives
2 large eggs and 1 egg white, lightly beaten
sea salt and black pepper

Heat the olive oil in a frying pan and throw in the garlic to flavour the oil. Add the courgette, spinach and chives and sauté for 3 minutes. Transfer the cooked vegetables to a plate or dish.

Return the pan to the heat and pour in the beaten eggs. Once the egg has set underneath, remove from the heat. Flip the omelette over and remove from the heat. Leave in the pan for 2 minutes to cook further.

Slide the cooked omelette onto a plate and spoon the vegetables over one half of the omelette. Fold the omelette over the vegetables and sprinkle with salt and pepper.

Consume.

The Food Plan

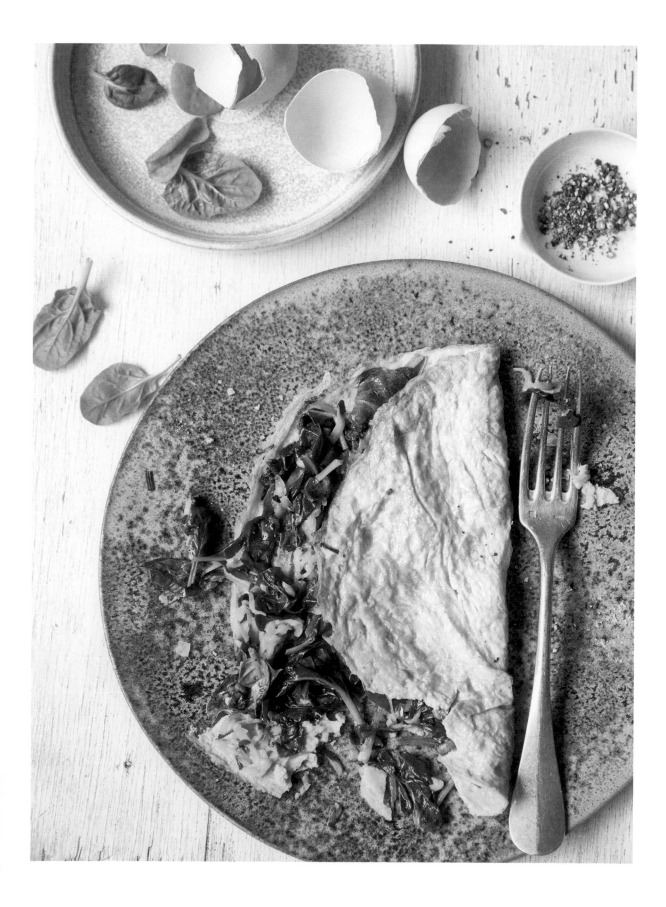

THE GREEN BOSS SMOOTHIE

I am a massive fan of green smoothies over juices. The benefit of a smoothie is that you don't lose the fibrous content of the vegetable or fruit like you do in a juice – the fibre has multiple benefits to the body and so shouldn't be left out. If you want an energy kick, add a teaspoon of matcha tea to the mix.

100ml unsweetened almond milk, or other nut milk alternative
100ml water
35g baby spinach
½ frozen banana
20g scoop vanilla protein powder
½ tsp ground cinnamon
4 ice cubes

Add the liquids to the blender first, then add the rest of the ingredients. Blend, consume and enjoy.

THE PRE-WORKOUT COFFEE DELICIOUSNESS SHAKE

This is the perfect option for those of you, like me, who cannot fathom training on an empty stomach, but need a quick-digesting breakfast that will also spike your energy levels (thank you, coffee). Coffee is a stimulant and it will kick-start your sympathetic nervous system (fight or flight mode). This is a good thing pre workout, as it will provide you with some intense energy and willpower for the training, but it's not such a good thing post workout. When you've finished a training session you actually want to calm the sympathetic nervous system down, stimulating the parasympathetic (rest and digest): think deep breathing and rehydration with water.

2 shots of espresso (or filtered coffee)
1 frozen banana
50ml oat or rice milk
20g scoop vanilla protein powder
5 ice cubes

Put all the ingredients into a blender and blend until creamy and smooth, adding the teeniest bit of water if it has trouble blending.

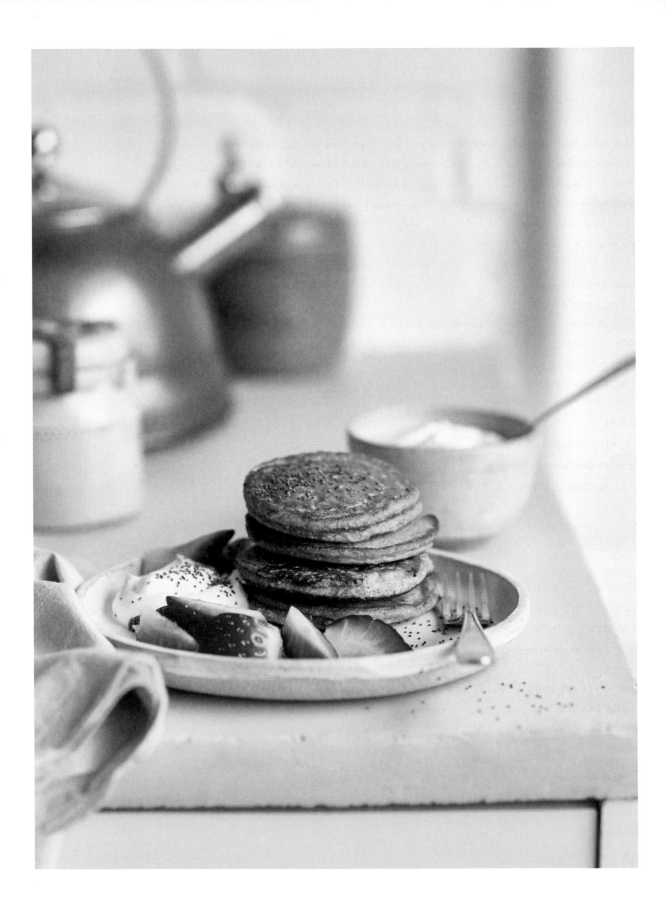

EASIER-THAN-YOU-THINK PROTEIN PANCAKES

Not only is this dish a favourite of mine on a Sunday morning when an omelette just doesn't feel festive enough, it's also my go-to when I know that I will be leaving the house early, forced to consume breakfast on the hop (don't judge me, we can't all meditate over our breakfast every day). I make the pancakes the night before, allow them to cool and wrap them in foil to be devoured the next morning (without the yoghurt – obviously!).

1 banana, chopped
2 large egg whites
15g protein powder (any flavour you like)
50g rolled oats
1 tsp ground cinnamon
1 tsp butter or coconut oil

to serve
a dollop of low-fat organic Greek yoghurt or coconut yoghurt
5 strawberries
½ tsp poppy seeds (optional, but delicious)

Place the banana, egg whites, protein powder, oats and cinnamon in a blender and whizz for a few seconds until smooth.

Melt the butter or coconut oil in a frying pan and swirl it around the pan to coat the base evenly. Add enough batter to the pan to make a palm-sized pancake and cook for about 1–1½ minutes, until set underneath. Flip and cook the other side, pressing it down slightly as it rises.

Remove from the pan and keep warm while you make more pancakes with the remaining batter (you should get at least 3 from the mixture), scraping out the bowl to make use of every last bit.

Serve with the yoghurt and strawberries, sprinkled with poppy seeds if you like.

VERTUEOUS VEGGIE BOX

Preparing the food you're going to eat for the day is key to staying on track (and is also way cheaper). However, Sunday night 'weekly food preps' are quite boring and they often take the passion out of our food, leaving us feeling lacklustre and eventually uninspired. When this happens, somehow on a subconscious level we can start to label 'healthy' food as 'boring, unloved, obligatory' food. That is the last thing I want to happen to you on this 28-day journey, so you will only ever prepare your salad on the night before or morning of lunchtime consumption, putting as much love as possible into each meal.

All you have to do is:

1. Prepare your protein and wrap it in foil or cling film, or pack it in a container.

2. Fill your lunchbox with the fruit and veg. (Hold off on adding the protein; you'll add it later.)

3. Make your dressing in a small, sealable jar to take separately.

4. When hunger strikes, pour over your dressing, add in your protein, give it a mix (or shake with the lid back on) and, look at that – you've got yourself a delicious and nutritious salad.

All recipes serve one.

GREEN GREEK SALAD

Mediterranean food is both nourishing and refreshing. Cucumber has a high water content and is great at keeping the body hydrated while also providing it with some fibre. The added spinach, although definitely not an aspect of a traditional Greek salad – *signómi* **(translation: 'I'm sorry' in Greek) – bulks it out with a little more fibre and micronutrients.**

a portion of protein of your choice (see pages 59–61)
100g cucumber, diced
5 black Kalamata olives, pitted
½ red onion, finely sliced
10 cherry tomatoes, sliced
40g baby spinach
30g low-fat feta cheese

for the dressing
1 tsp balsamic vinegar
1 tbsp olive oil
1 tsp fresh oregano leaves
1 tsp fresh thyme leaves

Prepare your protein and wrap it in foil or cling film, or pack it in a container.

Fill your lunchbox with the rest of the salad ingredients. (Hold off on adding the protein; you'll add it later.)

Make your dressing in a small, sealable jar to take separately.

When hunger strikes, pour over your dressing, add in your protein and give it a mix (or shake it with the lid back on).

RED APPLE AND PUY LENTIL SALAD

Watercress is one of my favourite ingredients because it's tasty and high in vitamin C (which is required for collagen synthesis – keeping our skin, nails, hair and all connective tissue healthy). It's also high in vitamin A, as well as minerals such as calcium and manganese. The red apple gives this salad some sweetness and the sugar snaps some crunch. I cook batches of lentils and store them in the fridge for a week.

a portion of protein of your choice (see pages 59–61)
2 handfuls of watercress
1 red apple, cored and finely chopped
8 sugar snap peas, halved lengthways
50g cooked Puy lentils

for the dressing
1 tsp balsamic vinegar
1 tbsp olive oil

Prepare your protein and wrap it in foil or cling film, or pack it in a container.

Fill your lunchbox with the rest of the salad ingredients. (Hold off on adding the protein; you'll add it later.)

Make your dressing in a small, sealable jar to take separately.

When hunger strikes, pour over your dressing, add in your protein and give it a mix (or shake it with the lid back on).

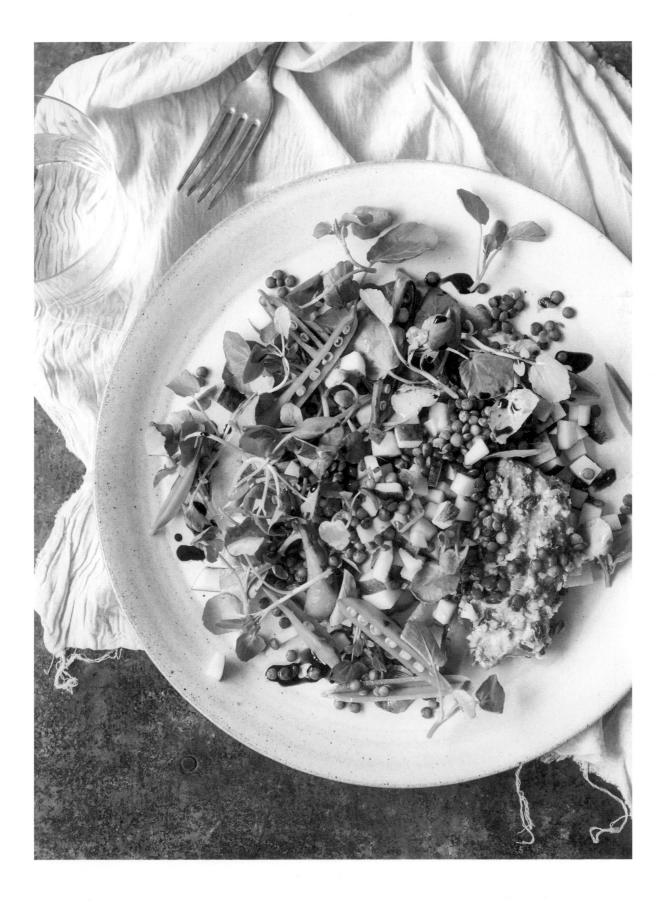

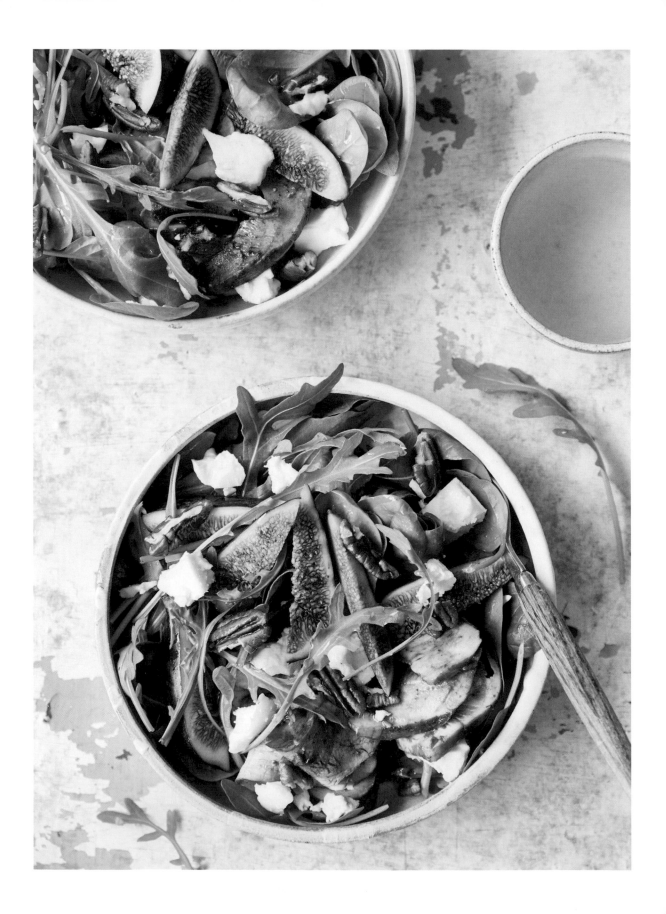

FIG, PECAN AND FETA SALAD

If you're not a 'salad person', I think this combination might change your mind (and taste buds). I have converted many avid salad haters with this alliance of flavours. It's important to choose your figs wisely as they don't ripen after picking, so make sure you buy fruit with a deep purple colour and an unbroken skin.

a portion of protein of your choice (see pages 59–61)
40g baby spinach
20g rocket
5 pecan nuts
1 fresh fig, sliced
50g low-fat feta cheese

for the dressing
juice of ½ lemon
½ tsp honey
1 tbsp olive oil

Prepare your protein and wrap it in foil or cling film, or pack it in a container.

Fill your lunchbox with the rest of the salad ingredients. (Hold off on adding the protein; you'll add it later.)

Make your dressing in a small, sealable jar to take separately.

When hunger strikes, pour over your dressing, add in your protein and give it a mix (or shake it with the lid back on).

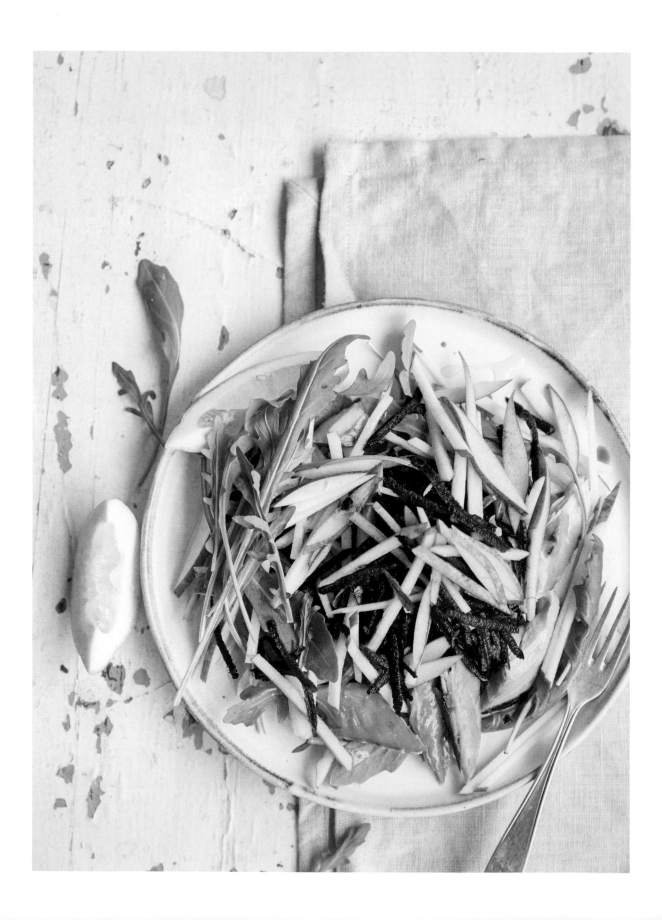

CRUNCHY RAW BEETROOT SALAD WITH PEAR

I recognise that beetroot is a bit of a love/hate kind of vegetable, but when matched with pear it tastes fresh and fruity. This is absolutely one of my favourite salads. One study has suggested that because of its betaine content, drinking beetroot juice post workout may reduce muscle soreness. Either way, it contains various vitamins and minerals that will support your body, so embrace the beet.

a portion of protein of your choice (see pages 59–61)
1 medium raw beetroot, washed and grated
1 pear, thinly sliced then cut into matchsticks
40g rocket

for the dressing
juice of ½ lemon
1 tbsp olive oil

Prepare your protein and wrap it in foil or cling film, or pack it in a container.

Fill your lunchbox with the rest of the salad ingredients. (Hold off on adding the protein; you'll add it later.)

Make your dressing in a small, sealable jar to take separately.

When hunger strikes, pour over your dressing, add in your protein and give it a mix (or shake it with the lid back on).

POMEGRANATE AND AVOCADO SALAD

At family gatherings my mother would make huge bowls of this summer salad and as I child I was always caught rummaging through the bowl in an effort to steal all the avocado (much to the dismay of my cousins). Children eat very intuitively and I think it's interesting that I was drawn towards good fats, supporting the development of a growing body and brain.

a portion of protein of your choice (see pages 59–61)
80g rocket
50g cooked, cooled runner beans (in chunks; steamed for 8–10 minutes
  or boiled for 5–8 minutes)
seeds of ½ pomegranate
½ avocado, sliced

for the dressing
40g raspberries blended with 2 tsp olive oil
1 tsp fresh thyme leaves

Prepare your protein and wrap it in foil or cling film, or pack it in a container.

Fill your lunchbox with the rest of the salad ingredients. (Hold off on adding the protein; you'll add it later.)

Make your dressing in a small, sealable jar to take separately.

When hunger strikes, pour over your dressing, add in your protein and give it a mix (or shake it with the lid back on).

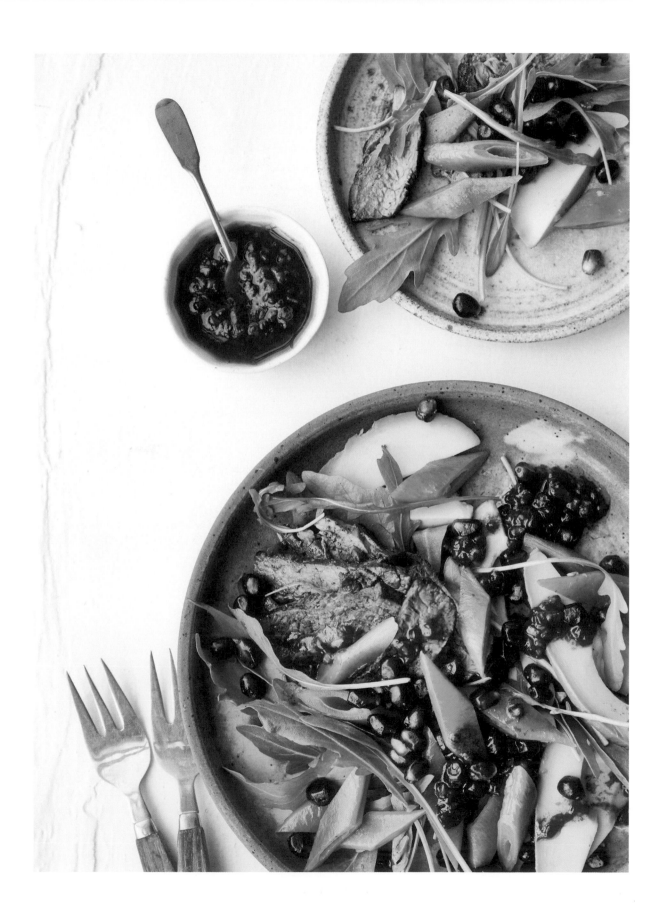

STRAWBERRY AND CUCUMBER SALAD WITH WATERCRESS

The first time I tried strawberry and balsamic vinegar together was actually in a dessert and from that moment I was hooked. I love this salad because it holds so many interesting flavours and textures (and obviously nutrients too!).

a portion of protein of your choice (see pages 59–61)
100g cucumber, chopped or sliced
100g strawberries, quartered
80g watercress

for the dressing
1 tsp balsamic vinegar
2 tsp olive oil

Prepare your protein and wrap it in foil or cling film, or pack it in a container.

Fill your lunchbox with the rest of the salad ingredients. (Hold off on adding the protein; you'll add it later.)

Make your dressing in a small, sealable jar to take separately.

When hunger strikes, pour over your dressing, add in your protein and give it a mix (or shake it with the lid back on).

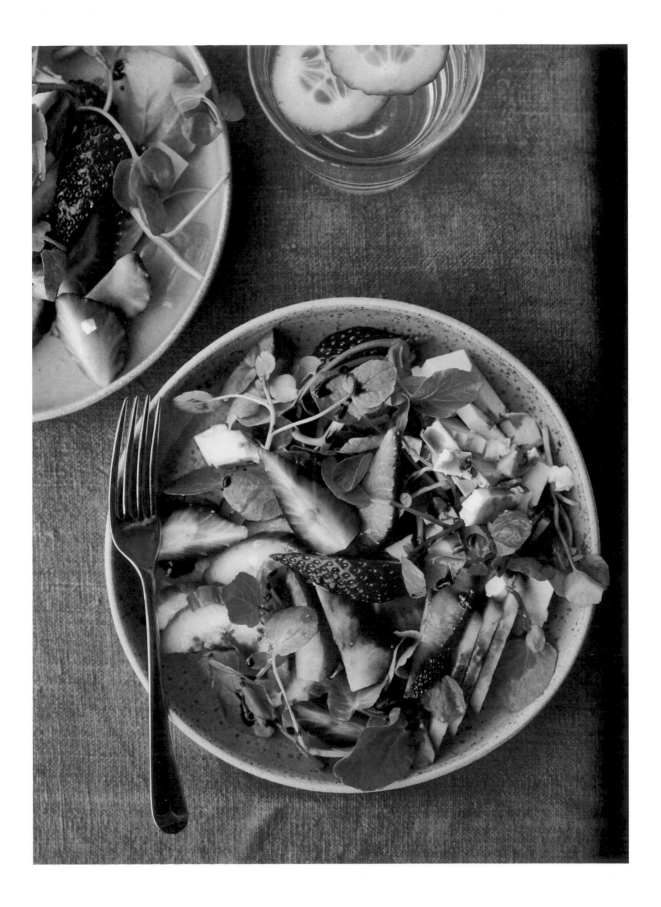

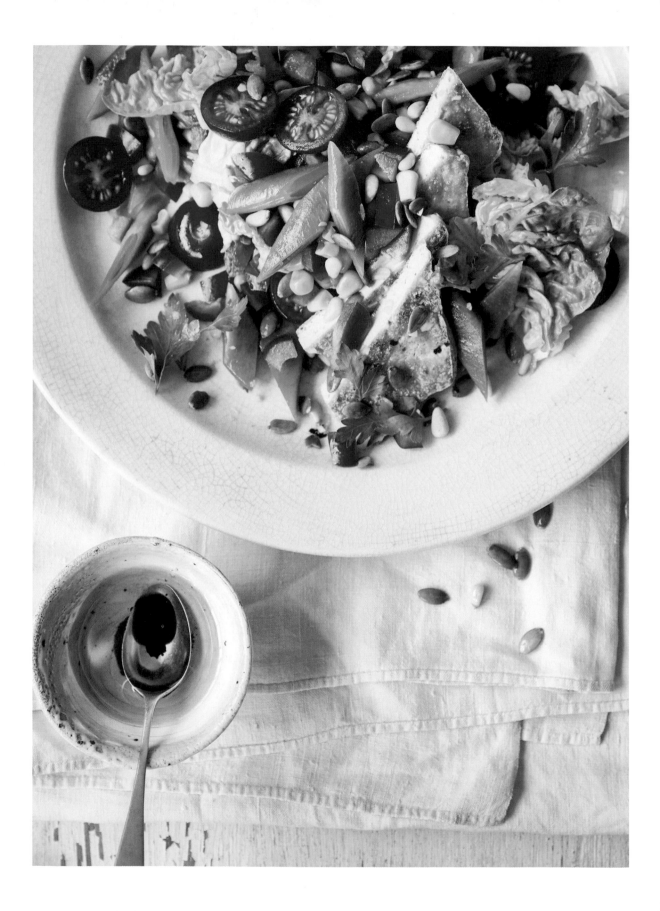

GARDEN SALAD

While this salad contains a lot of vitamin-dense ingredients, can we all just take a moment to celebrate pumpkin seeds? These little guys are high in zinc (a key player in sustaining a healthy immune system) as well as magnesium (which has been shown to help reduce anxiety and also improve sleep). While it may seem like you're having an insignificant amount, every little bit counts. This salad included.

a portion of protein of your choice (see pages 59–61)
50g cooked, cooled runner beans
  (in chunks; steamed for 8–10 minutes or boiled for 5–8 minutes)
75g cherry tomatoes, halved
50g canned sweetcorn (drained weight)
a sprig of parsley, chopped
1 small red pepper (capsicum), deseeded and sliced
10g pine nuts
10g pumpkin seeds
70g Romaine lettuce leaves

for the dressing
1 tbsp olive oil
1 tsp balsamic vinegar

Prepare your protein and wrap it in foil or cling film, or pack it in a container.

Fill your lunchbox with the rest of the salad ingredients. (Hold off on adding the protein; you'll add it later.)

Make your dressing in a small, sealable jar to take separately.

When hunger strikes, pour over your dressing, add in your protein and give it a mix (or shake it with the lid back on).

BE THE MASTER OF YOUR OWN DESTINY (AND SALAD)

I recognise that you're not always going to want to follow a plan. I also recognise the benefit of keeping creativity as an element within your food preparation to maintain interest and be able to use your own inspiration. You'll be on this plan for 28 days and sometimes you will want to play with different greens and ingredients.

Here's how to design your own salad following just a few of my guidelines:
- You can never eat too many leafy greens – feel free to go crazy with different leaves.
- Have no more than one serving of the 'sweet' column per salad.
- Consume no more than one thumb-sized serving of nuts per salad.
- Stay away from processed dressings and instead make your own (stick to no more than 1 tbsp oil per salad).
- Don't forget to add your serving of protein.

LEAF BASE	CRUNCH	SWEET	SOMETHING SOFT	NUTTY
Baby spinach	Cucumber	Apples	Avocado	Cashews
Cabbage	Carrots	Blueberries	Low-fat cheese	Pine nuts
Lettuce	Sprouts	Mango	Olives	Hemp seeds
Pea shoots	Courgette (zucchini)	Melon	Tomato	Pumpkin seeds
Rocket	Pepper (capsicum)	Papaya		Sunflower seeds
Watercress		Strawberries		Toasted almonds
				Walnuts

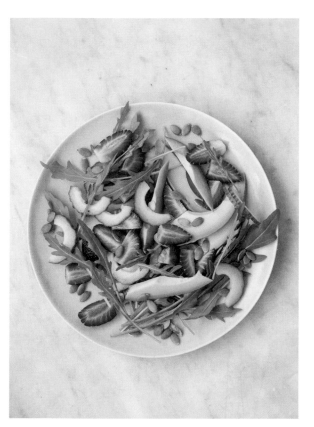 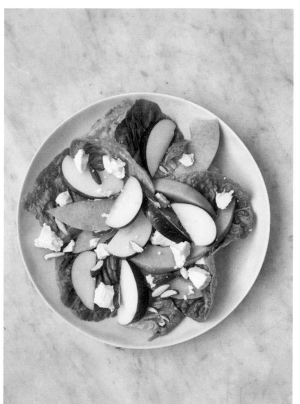

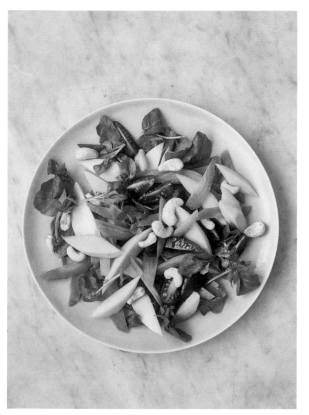 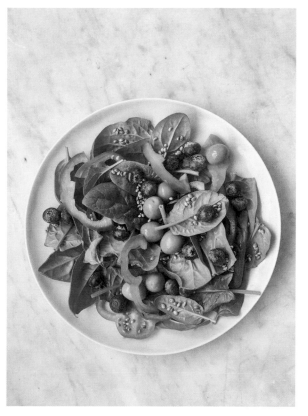

DINNER

These meals differ, depending on the type of training you have completed on each day. On your weight-dominant days (workouts VM1 and 2), you're going to be consuming a '**Booty-full Bowl**' which includes more starch-based vegetables to replenish muscle glycogen that has been depleted from high repetition resistance training.

On cardio days (VM3) you'll be consuming a big phat bowl of **Lean Greens** packed with energising micronutrients to nourish your body and brain.

Booty-full Bowls (to be consumed on VM1 and VM2 workout days): pages 232–45.

Lean Greens (to be consumed on VM3 workout and rest days): pages 246–53.

The dinner recipes have been doubled to serve two. This is to accommodate hungry friends and lovers, or if you're dining alone simply to save time, so you can store them away as leftovers.

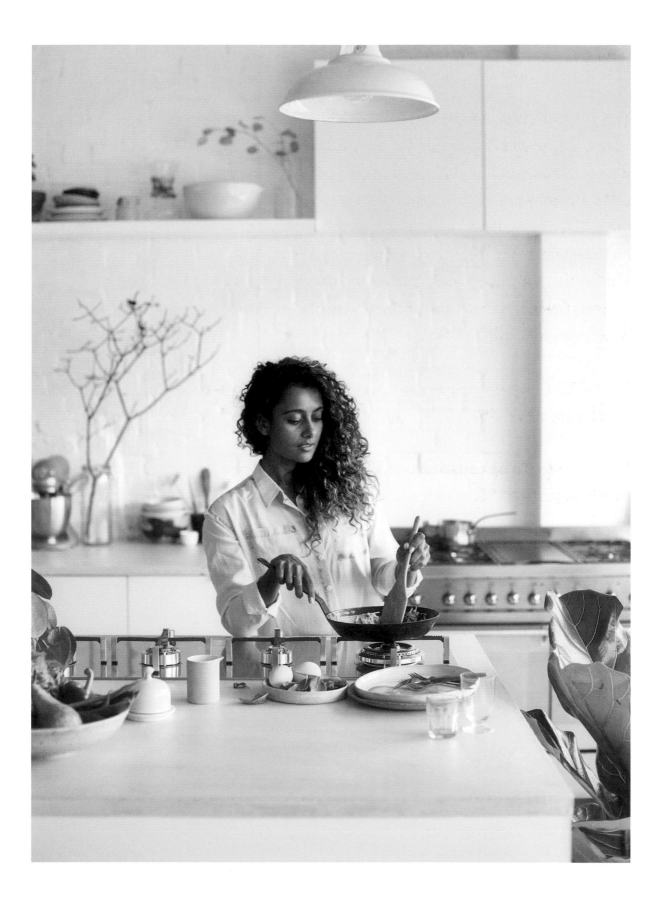

STIR-FRIED GREENS WITH SOBA NOODLES

I love a crispy stir-fry and I also love soba noodles – they are made from buckwheat which is low in calories and high in fibre and protein. Buckwheat also contains a decent serving of manganese (a trace mineral that helps the body to form connective tissue and also supports carbohydrate metabolisation). From a taste perspective, these are delicious hot or cold and are super easy to prepare. Be sure not to overcook your veggies; soggy stir-fries are uninspiring and sad.

100g soba noodles
1 tbsp olive oil
1 tbsp chopped ginger
1 tsp crushed garlic
1 small onion, finely chopped
160g mangetout
20g spring onions, finely sliced
120g carrots, cut into fine ribbons using a swivel peeler
½ chilli, deseeded and sliced
a sprig of coriander, chopped
a portion of cooked protein of your choice (see pages 59–61) per serving

for the sauce
1 tbsp soy sauce
1 tbsp water

Cook the soba noodles according to the packet instructions, then drain.

Meanwhile, heat the olive oil in a wok and add the ginger, garlic and onion. Cook until the onion becomes transparent, then add the mangetout, spring onions, carrots and chilli and cook, stirring, for 2 minutes.

Mix the soy sauce with the water and add to the vegetables. Stir and immediately take off the heat. Add the noodles to serving bowls, then add the vegetables, sprinkle over the coriander and serve with your chosen protein.

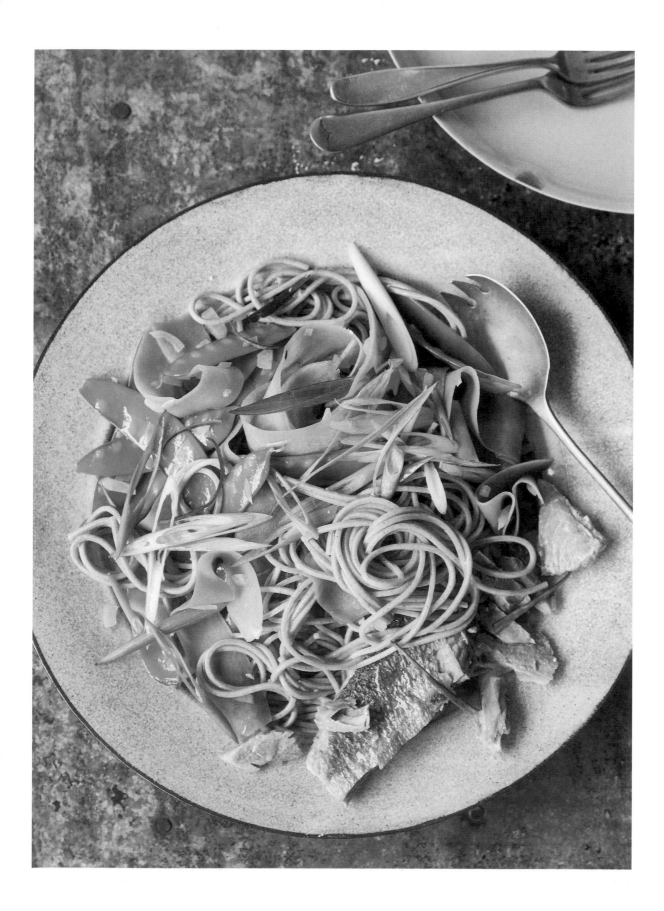

KALE AND QUINOA BOWL WITH CHILLI AND CORIANDER

Quinoa is a complete protein, so it contains all nine essential amino acids. The kale adds some green power to the mix: it's high in fibre, vitamin K and has more iron per calorie than beef! This bowl will leave you feeling nourished and satisfied.

85g quinoa
170ml water
1 tbsp olive oil
1 garlic clove, very finely chopped
100g kale, chopped
a handful of coriander leaves
½ chilli, finely chopped (optional)

Put the quinoa and water into a pan and bring to the boil. Reduce the heat and simmer for about 15–20 minutes, until the quinoa is cooked and all the water is absorbed. Remove from the heat and set aside.

Heat the olive oil in a wok or frying pan, add the garlic and kale and sauté over a low heat until the kale wilts. Stir in the cooked quinoa and serve immediately, topped with the coriander, and chilli if using.

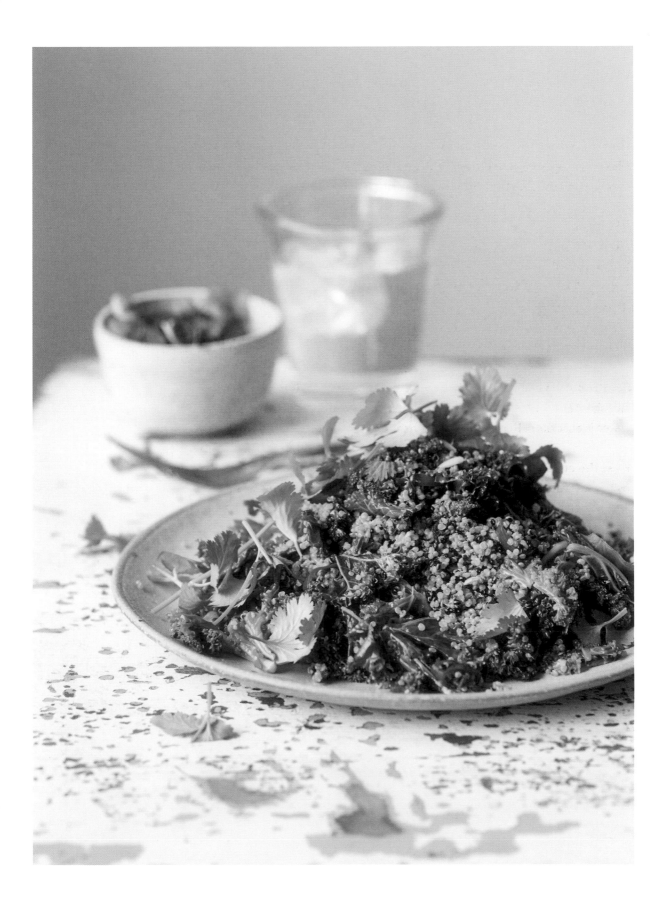

TACO BOWL

This bowl is awesome because it becomes a complete protein with the combination of beans and rice. This is actually my favourite of the Booty-full Bowls because it's so filling and comforting, partly because of its nutrient density. Don't worry if you feel overwhelmed by the number of ingredients on this list – it will be worth it and you will be extremely nourished.

120g canned kidney beans (drained weight)
160g lettuce, finely shredded
125g canned sweetcorn (drained weight)
½ avocado, sliced
a handful of tortilla chips, slightly crushed

for the salsa
1 medium tomato, finely chopped
1 small red onion, finely diced
1 tsp finely chopped garlic
a sprig of coriander, finely chopped
juice of 1 lime
1 tbsp extra virgin olive oil
a pinch of sea salt

for the rice
100g basmati rice
500ml water
½ tsp Mexican spice mix (or use
    a pinch each of cayenne pepper,
    cumin, paprika, garlic salt and
    black pepper)

Put all the salsa ingredients into a large bowl, mix well and set aside.

Put the rice into a large pan with the water and spice mix. Bring to the boil then turn the heat down and simmer for 10–12 minutes. Remove from the heat and give it a stir with a wooden spoon. If it's still too watery, replace the lid and allow it to sit for 5–10 minutes.

When the rice is nearly cooked, heat the kidney beans either in the microwave, or in a frying pan with a tiny dash of water.

Place the lettuce in the bottom of two bowls. Fluff the rice with a fork and divide it between them. Divide the kidney beans and stir them through the rice, then top each bowl with the sweetcorn, avocado, salsa and tortilla chips.

The Food Plan

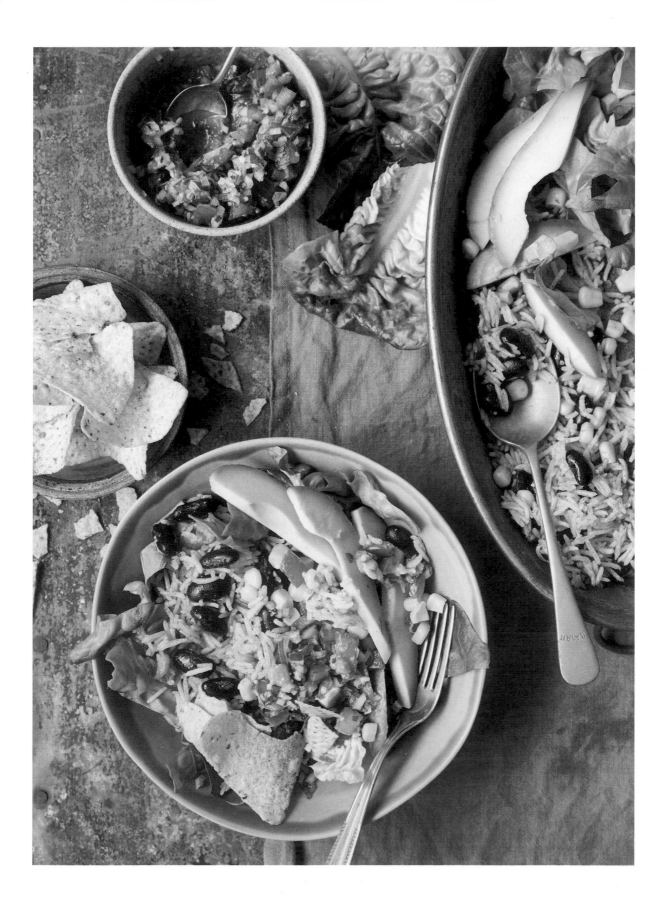

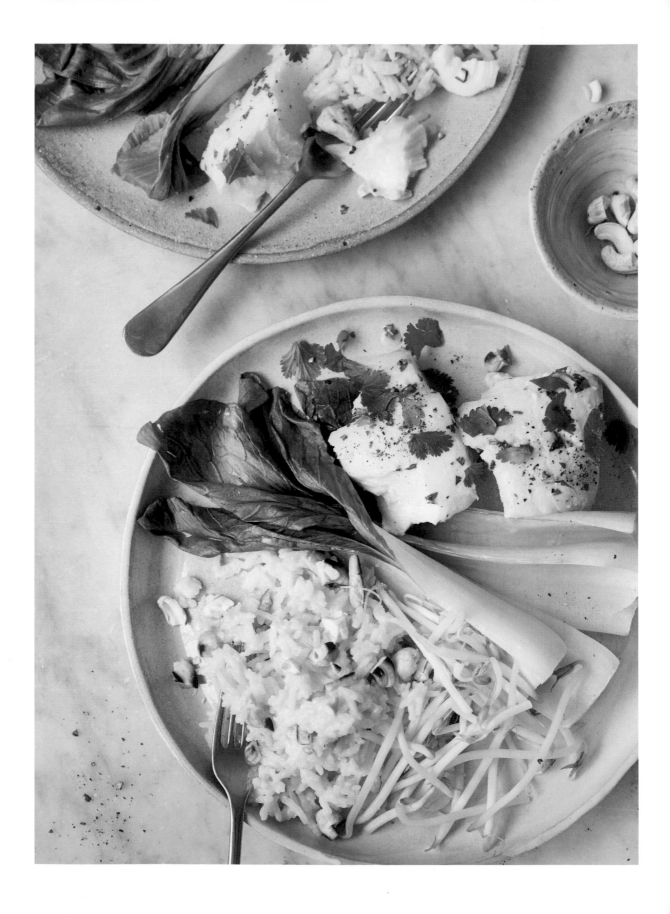

STEAMED VEGGIES WITH GINGER AND COCONUT RICE

I'm quite obsessed with coconut rice – having an islander mum will turn you into a coconut lover. While it does raise the fat content of this meal, I personally think the taste alone makes it worth it.

250g pak choi
a handful of bean sprouts
20g dry-roasted cashew nuts
a portion of cooked protein of your choice
  (see pages 59–61) per serving

for the rice
100g basmati rice
a pinch of salt
235ml water
235ml coconut milk
1 tsp grated ginger

for the sauce
2 tbsp soy sauce
1 tsp honey

Put the rice in a large pan with the salt, water, coconut milk and ginger. Bring to the boil then turn down and simmer for 10–12 minutes. Remove from the heat and give it a stir with a wooden spoon. If it's still too watery, replace the lid and allow it to sit for 5–10 minutes.

Once the rice is almost done, steam the pak choi for 4 minutes, ensuring it does not overcook.

In a small bowl, mix the soy sauce with the honey, stirring vigorously.

Fluff the rice up and divide between two bowls, place the pak choi, bean sprouts and cashews on top and spoon over the sauce. Serve with your chosen protein.

MUM'S TURMERIC AND HONEY-ROASTED SWEET POTATOES WITH MANGETOUT

My very fit and healthy mum is part Fijian part Indian and she was using turmeric way before it was trendy. In fact she basically put turmeric in everything, this recipe being my favourite of all. Turmeric is fat-soluble, so in order for you to reap its benefits you must consume it with fat (the piperine in black pepper can also help to raise its bioavailability). I warn you that this dish is moreish so if you're dining alone, make sure you put one serving to the side before you sit down to yours.

1 tbsp coconut oil
1 tbsp honey
175g sweet potato, cut into 2.5cm chunks
1 tsp ground cinnamon
1 tsp ground turmeric
200g mangetout
black pepper
a portion of cooked protein of your choice (see pages 59–61) per serving

Preheat the oven to 200°C/gas 6.

Heat the coconut oil and honey together over a gentle heat in a small pan, just until melted. Spread the sweet potatoes out in a baking dish. Add the melted coconut oil and honey with the cinnamon and turmeric, and mix thoroughly, making sure the sweet potato pieces are well coated. Add black pepper to taste.

Bake in the oven for 25 minutes, or until cooked through and slightly crispy.

About 5 minutes before the potatoes are ready, bring a large pan of water to the boil and place a metal colander on top. Once the water is boiling, check the colander is not touching the water and put the mangetout inside. Cover with a lid and steam for 3 minutes.

Remove the sweet potato from the oven and allow to cool slightly. Drain any excess liquid from the mangetout and spoon onto plates, with the sweet potato. Serve with your chosen protein.

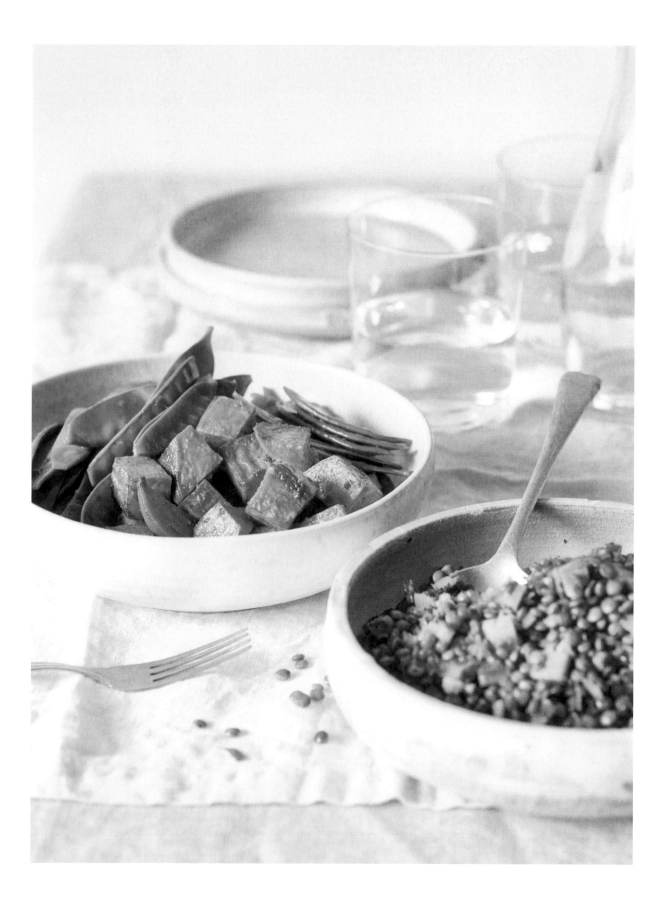

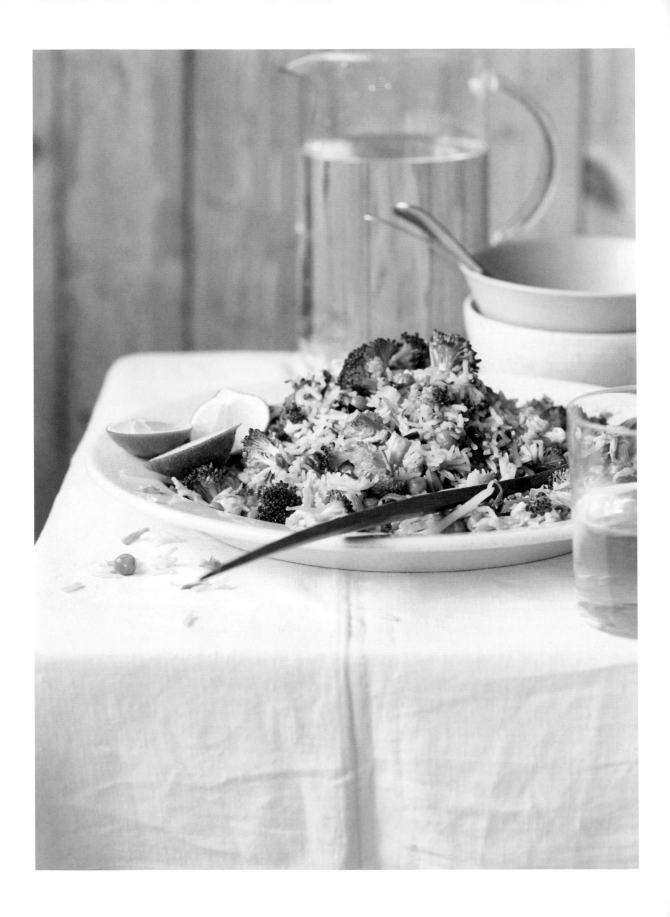

FRIED RICE FOR PHATTIES

This dish is pretty hot and tempting, hence its name. It's also another great way to use leftovers. I don't mind if you add any more vegetables that you might have left over from your lunch or an earlier cook. The only problem with fried rice is that it can be so delicious that you end up eating two portions of it. Otherwise you will find yourself fork deep in a second serving. Fried rice doesn't keep well so if you're dining alone, make half the quantity and then make it again later in the week.

1 tbsp coconut oil
1 tsp crushed garlic
1 tsp grated ginger
2 spring onions, finely chopped
120g carrots, grated
100g courgette (zucchini), grated
100g red cabbage, chopped
100g broccoli, chopped
50g peas
a handful of bean sprouts
1 tbsp soy sauce

1 tsp honey
juice of 1 lime
2 medium eggs, beaten
a portion of cooked protein of your
    choice (see pages 59–61) per serving

for the rice
100g basmati rice
500ml water
a pinch of sea salt

Put the rice in a large pan with the water and salt. Bring to the boil then turn down and simmer for 10–12 minutes. Remove from the heat and give it a stir with a wooden spoon. If it's still too watery, replace the lid and allow it to sit for 5–10 minutes.

Melt the coconut oil in a large frying pan or wok, throw in the garlic, ginger and spring onions and sauté until fragrant, then add the carrots, courgette, red cabbage, broccoli, peas and bean sprouts, and mix well. Keep stirring over the heat until everything is almost cooked.

Throw in the cooked rice and mix well.

In a small bowl, mix the soy sauce with the honey and lime juice, pour over the rice and vegetables and stir to mix.

Make a little gap in the pan to the side of the rice and vegetables and pour in the beaten egg. Leave to cook a little, then stir it through the rest of the rice. Serve with your chosen protein.

ROAST VEGGIES WITH ROSEMARY AND GARLIC

I think everyone has been handed down a slightly different way of doing a roast dish. My nan used to use duck fat on all the vegetables, while my mum coated everything in coconut oil and curry leaves. This recipe is very simple and foolproof, however if you like certain herbs or would prefer to use a different oil, go ahead – just aim to stick to the same amounts.

115g parsnip, cut into long chunks (quarters if from 1 parsnip)
150g baby carrots
1 small red onion, peeled and quartered
160g baby new potatoes
1 small red pepper (capsicum), deseeded and quartered
1 small green pepper (capsicum), deseeded and quartered
1 tsp finely chopped garlic
a sprig of rosemary, leaves picked
½ tsp dried oregano
1 tbsp olive oil
a portion of cooked protein of your choice (see pages 59–61) per serving

Preheat the oven to 200°C/gas 6.

Spread the parsnip, carrots, onion, potatoes and peppers out in a baking dish.

Combine the garlic, rosemary, oregano and olive oil in a small bowl and drizzle over the veggies. Mix thoroughly and bake in the oven for 30–35 minutes, turning them halfway through cooking.

Serve with your chosen protein.

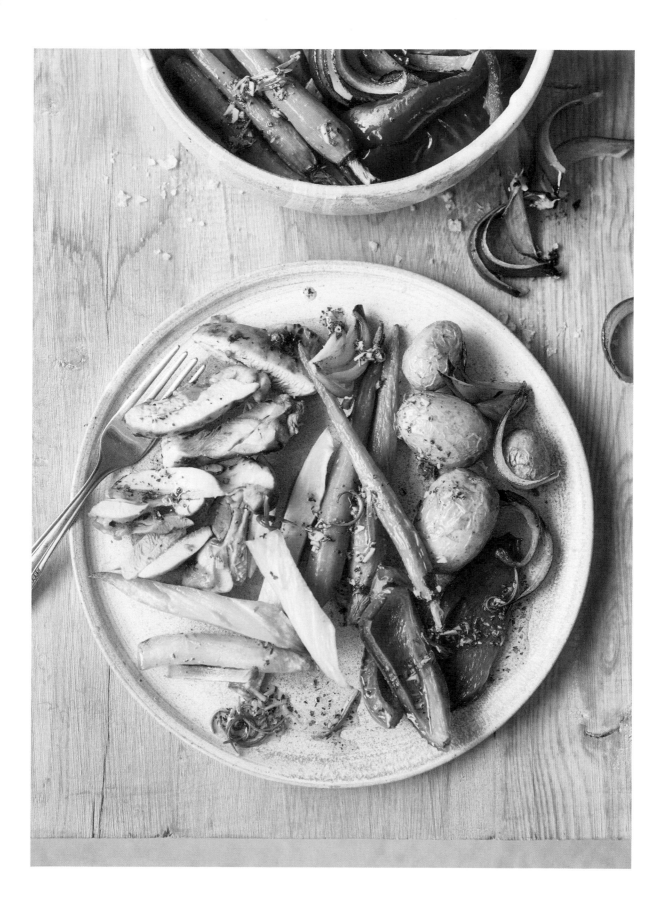

ASIAN STIR-FRIED GREENS AND CARROT

This is my go-to dish when I've had one of those naughty, 'didn't-eat-enough-greens' kind of days because it's quick, easy and very tasty. Pak choi is part of the cruciferous vegetable family. Aside from the other awesome vitamins and minerals contained in cruciferous vegetables, 170g (a cup) of pak choi can provide us with half our RDI of vitamin C.

1 tsp olive oil
1 garlic clove, crushed
1 tsp grated ginger
250g pak choi, washed and halved
2 carrots, cut into fine ribbons using a swivel peeler
1 tsp sesame seeds
a portion of cooked protein (see pages 59–61) per serving

for the sauce
1 tbsp soy sauce
2 tsp lime juice
1 tsp honey

For the sauce, mix the soy sauce, lime juice and honey together in a small bowl.

Heat a wok or large frying pan over a high heat. Swirl in the olive oil and add the garlic and ginger. Stir until sizzling and fragrant.

Add the pak choi, stir-fry for 1–2 minutes then add the carrot ribbons and pak choi leaves.

Pour in the sauce and cook, stirring and tossing the vegetables frequently, for about 3–5 minutes until the pak choi leaves are wilted and the stalks are tender. Sprinkle the sesame seeds on top and serve with your chosen protein.

The Food Plan

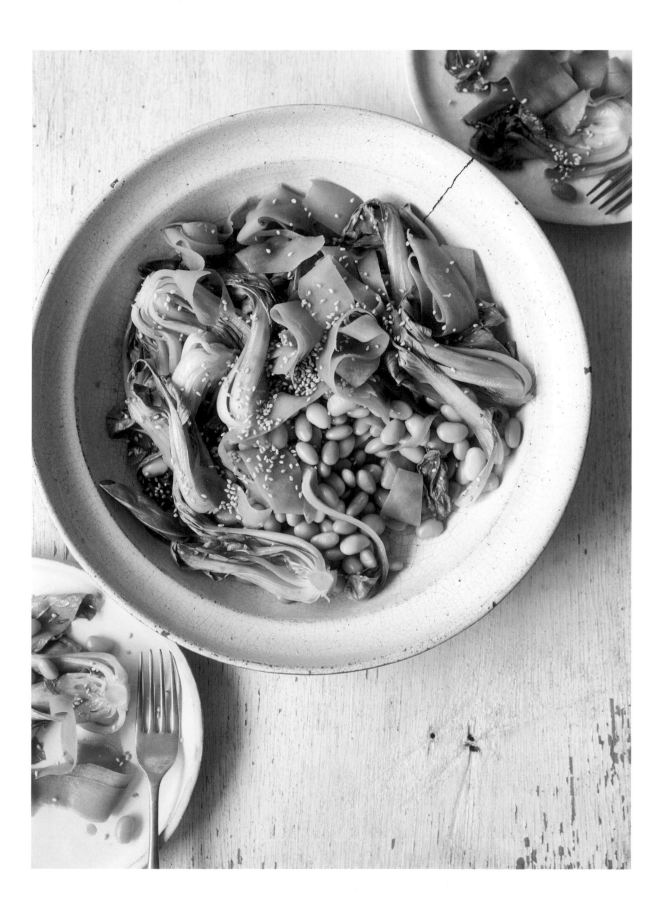

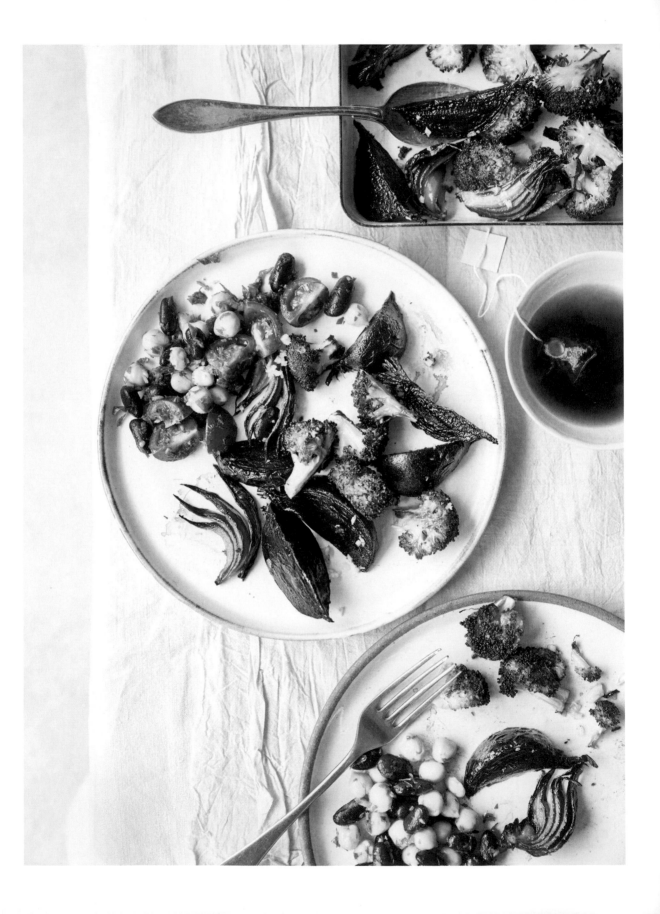

ROASTED BROCCOLI AND BEETROOT

This is such a beautiful and heart-warming dish. Roasting vegetables can often raise the bioavailability of certain nutrients within them. It also stops nutrients from leaching out into water as they would in boiling.

200g broccoli, separated into florets
2 small raw beetroot (unpeeled), washed and quartered
1 tbsp olive oil
1 small red onion, sliced
1 garlic clove, crushed
a pinch of sea salt
a portion of cooked protein of your choice (see pages 59–61) per serving

Preheat the oven to 200°C/gas 6 and line a baking tray with baking parchment.

In a medium bowl, toss the broccoli florets and beetroot quarters in the olive oil.

Transfer to the baking tray, add the onion and garlic, and spread the vegetables out evenly in a single layer.

Sprinkle with the salt and roast for 40 minutes, or until the broccoli is browned and the beetroot is soft. Drizzle any oil and cooking juices from the tray on top and serve with your chosen protein.

CHILLI STIR-FRIED KALE

If you think you don't like kale because you've been subjected to one of those awful kale smoothies or have only ever had it steamed, then I don't blame you, I wouldn't like it either. However, cooked in butter it is extremely delicious; the kale absorbs the butter like a sponge and what you're left with is a flavoursome cruciferous vegetable. Vegans can use coconut oil instead, which will still give buttery results.

1 tbsp butter
1 tsp finely chopped garlic
150g kale, roughly chopped
½ chilli, deseeded and chopped
seeds of ½ pomegranate
a portion of cooked protein of your choice (see pages 59–61) per serving

Melt the butter in a wok or large frying pan. Add the garlic and sauté very briefly until fragrant, about 30 seconds at the most.

Throw in the kale and cook for 5–7 minutes, until almost cooked, stirring frequently.

Add the chilli and cook for another minute.

Serve topped with the pomegranate seeds, with your chosen protein.

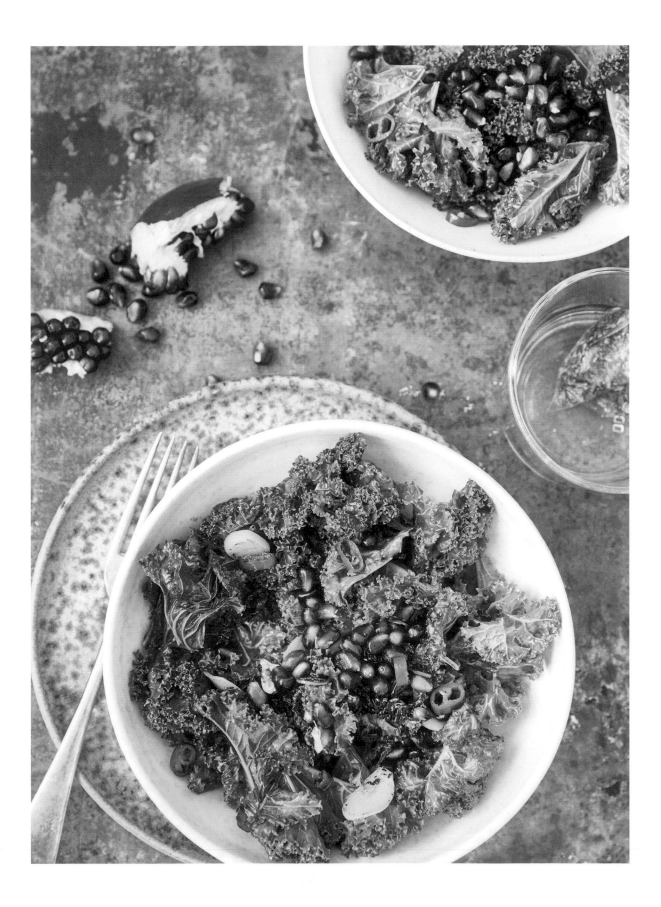

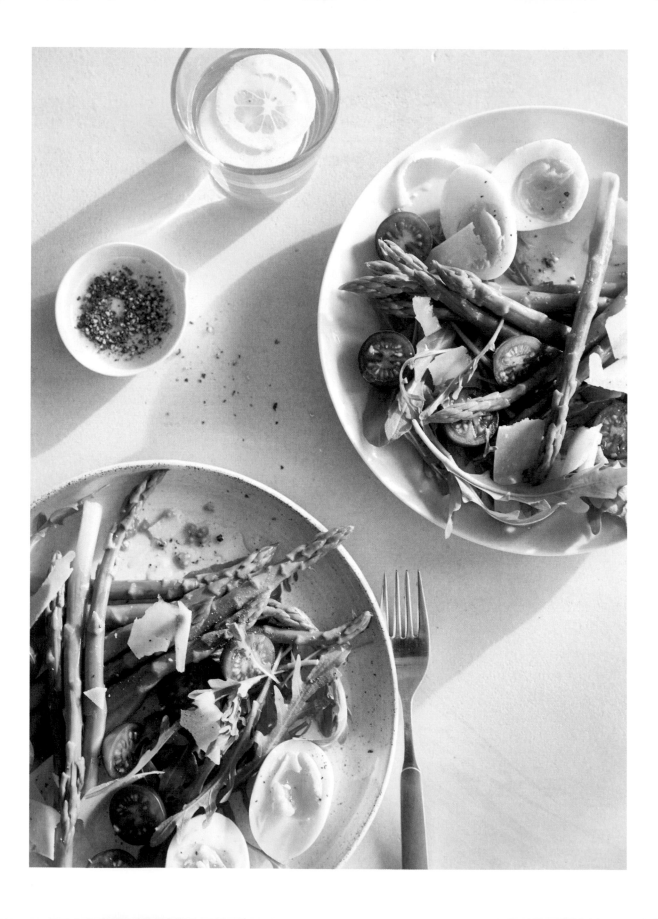

WARM ASPARAGUS SALAD

While I personally love my asparagus dripping in butter or egg yolk, it also works really well in this salad. Asparagus can provide us with around 15 per cent of our RDI of vitamin A, as well as 11 per cent of our recommended iron intake. Asparagus is a very seasonal vegetable and should really only be consumed in spring (in the UK). Eating seasonally helps you to obtain better, more nutritionally dense produce without too much negative human intervention (such as toxic pesticides and herbicides).

500g asparagus spears, halved crossways
  (you can use Tenderstem out of the asparagus season)
10 cherry tomatoes, halved
2 handfuls of rocket
1 tbsp olive oil
1 tsp grated Parmesan cheese (or vegan Parmesan)
a portion of cooked protein of your choice (see pages 59–61) per serving

Bring a large pan of water to the boil and place a metal colander on top. When the water is boiling (make sure it isn't touching the colander) place the asparagus inside the colander, cover with a lid and steam for 3–4 minutes until just tender. Remove, drain and allow to cool a little.

Put the cherry tomatoes and rocket onto serving plates, then place the warm asparagus on top.

Drizzle over the olive oil and sprinkle on the Parmesan. Serve with your chosen protein.

SMOOTHIES

To say that I am fond of smoothies would be a gross understatement. I love them in the deep, eternal and universal sense of the word. The reason being is that they taste great (if you have the right recipes), are easy to digest, can be a quick and easy source of protein and can curb that dessert craving that comes at the end of dinner – while still giving you a hit of micronutrients. You can absolutely have these at any time of the day, but I personally love to have a cooling smoothie at nighttime before bed or, if I'm in a hurry, I'll have one as a quick breakfast as all the smoothies here contain a minimum of 20g protein.

There are a few smoothie 'bowls' in my recipes – bowls tend to be thicker (yum) so that you can eat them with a spoon. Make sure your blender can handle them, though – sometimes cold ingredients will require a quick stir in between blends.

A note on protein powder – different protein powders contain different amounts of protein and have different-sized scoops. For every smoothie recipe there should be a minimum of 20g protein. Check the labelling and add more than one scoop if required.

All recipes serve one.

RASPBERRIES AND CREAM SMOOTHIE BOWL

New research suggests that raspberries (or a phytonutrient within them called rheosmin – aka raspberry ketone – may help in the prevention of obesity and fatty liver. They also taste great, so really it's a win-win situation.

1 frozen banana
150g low-fat plain yoghurt
10g (about ½ scoop) vanilla protein powder
50g raspberries
1 tsp vanilla powder or ½ tsp vanilla extract

Add all the ingredients to a blender, reserving a few raspberries for the top, and blend until creamy and smooth. You may need to stir in between bouts of blending to mix all the ingredients. Transfer to a bowl and top with extra berries to serve.

VANILLA 'ICE CREAM' SMOOTHIE

Sometimes it's just nice to keep things simple. Vanilla is underrated, in my opinion. It's an aphrodisiac, so bottoms-up, I guess.

1 frozen banana
50ml fortified unsweetened almond or oat milk,
  plus extra if needed
1 tsp vanilla powder
20g scoop vanilla protein powder
4 ice cubes

Add all the ingredients to a blender and blend until creamy and smooth, adding the teeniest bit of extra almond or oat milk if it has trouble blending. Enjoy immediately.

BLUEBERRY AND CARDAMOM SMOOTHIE BOWL

Cardamom is part of the same family as ginger and can help to alleviate digestive problems like an upset stomach. Good quality yoghurts contain probiotics, which play a role in so many functions within the body. In fact, there are some strains of gut flora that play a part in effective brain function. Fermented foods are also great for the gut.

50g frozen blueberries, plus a few extra for the top
150g low-fat plain yoghurt, or 70g coconut yoghurt
10g (about ½ scoop) vanilla protein powder
a teeny-tiny pinch of ground cardamom (too much will be overpowering)

Add all the ingredients to a blender and blend until creamy and smooth. You may need to stir in between bouts of blending to mix all the ingredients. Transfer to a bowl and top with extra berries to serve.

PAPAYA, GINGER AND CINNAMON SMOOTHIE

This smoothie tastes like a spicy island summer, and the ginger is extra soothing on the gut, as well as antibacterial. Cinnamon also helps to lower blood sugar – everyone wins with this smoothie.

100g ripe papaya, roughly cubed
½ tsp finely chopped ginger
1 tsp ground cinnamon
20g scoop vanilla protein powder
50–100ml plant-based milk of choice (add more or less
  for a more or less liquid smoothie; it's up to you)
4 ice cubes

Add all the ingredients to a blender and blend until creamy and smooth, adding the teeniest bit of water if it has trouble blending.

Enjoy immediately.

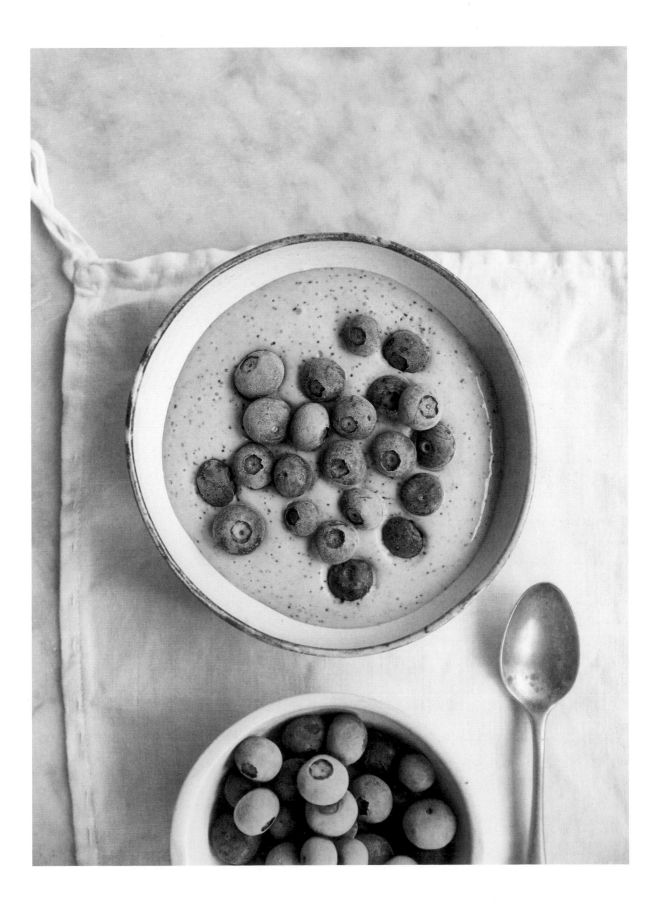

CHOCOLATE PEANUT BUTTER SMOOTHIE

This recipe is just a simple but audacious peanut butter smoothie. Peanut butter is so tasty and I think we should all just take a moment to appreciate it. However, I know that some of you will have that same appreciation for almond butter, so please feel free to use either in this recipe. Please make sure you choose nut butter that is made from sustainable palm oil or, better still, is completely free from palm oil (for ethical and environmental reasons).

1 small frozen banana
1 tsp organic peanut butter (or other sugar-free nut butter
  – Nutella doesn't count!)
150ml plant-based milk of choice
20g scoop vanilla protein powder
1 tbsp cacao powder
1 tsp ground cinnamon
4 ice cubes

Add all the ingredients to a blender and blend until creamy and smooth, adding the teeniest bit of water if it has trouble blending.

Smoothie Tips and Tricks:

1. Peel, slice and bag up bananas to freeze so that you can just whack them straight into your smoothie.

2. Make sure your ice containers are always full; there's nothing worse than a warm smoothie.

3. In my recipes I prefer to avoid dairy (see page 64 on veganism and reducing animal product intake to find out why) so I would love you to try a milk alternative. Almond milk can irritate some people's guts (like mine) so if that is the case, I would suggest you try switching it up with unsweetened oat or rice milk.

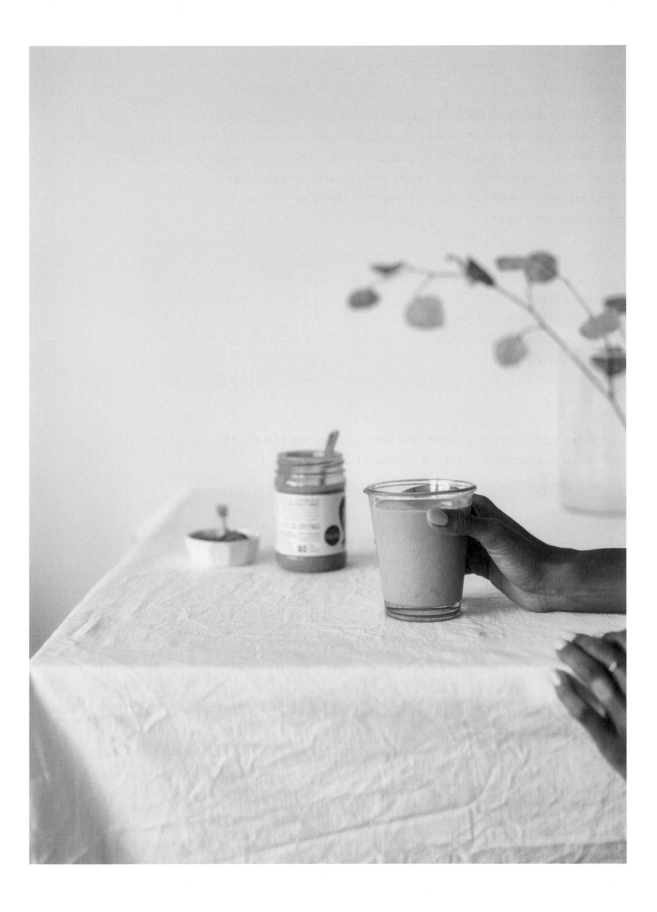

STAYING VERTUEOUS

WHAT TO DO AFTER THE 28-DAY RESET PLAN

Firstly, congratulations – and I don't mean for finishing, I mean for starting. By practising the Vertue Method 28-day reset plan you have chosen to prioritise your health, which really is more valuable than anything. The next step is allowing these principles to be integrated into your life beyond the 28 days, because ultimately that was the real intention for writing this book and the idea behind planning a 'reset'.

The absolute last thing I would recommend is to follow your full 28-day compliancy with a massive booze and processed food binge. There is no reason why you should stop doing what you have been doing for the last 28 days. In fact, research suggests that it takes a minimum of two months to change a habit, so it will be worth your effort to continue as you're already halfway there. I want to encourage you to embrace my nutritional and fitness philosophy in a way that will continue to enhance your vitality for life and fulfill your physical goals. My dream is that you begin to explore creative ways in which you can lift, lengthen and nourish yourself without the need for a recipe or a plan, because at the end of the day I do not want you living off 30 recipes for the rest of your life.

I don't vilify food groups – a glass of wine at the end of your week is not going to undo your results. Likewise, a slice of bread or some chocolate after dinner is, again, not going to undermine all of your hard work. You now know this because you've learned that food is simply made up of macronutrients (protein, carbohydrates and fat) and micronutrients (vitamins and minerals) and while it's best to make as many 'whole food' choices as possible, it is important for your soul that you enjoy the culinary pleasure of a 2005 Bordeaux coupled with a large bowl of home-made pasta. Rather than just trying to 'make a healthy choice', you now know how to make a choice that is both intuitive and educated. You will choose to eat an apple over a chocolate bar, not because I've told you it's healthier, but because you know that it will fuel your bodily systems, your day and your workout more effectively.

The point of the 28 days was to reset your approach to food, as well as your taste buds; to help you instil healthy habits that could be practised for the rest of your life, such as meditating and exercising daily, as well as eating intuitively, based on your body's needs. Ideally you will continue to maintain these practices, amending them as you see fit, to enhance your life and your body's ability to enjoy life.

Staying strong

After the 28 days of training, your body will have made some physiological adaptations that should have you stronger and more flexible. I recommend that you give yourself a few days off from training to relax and appreciate your hard work. Then, when the next Monday comes around, begin at the first workout – but this time aim to either lift heavier or lift more repetitions. This increase in weight or repetitions is called 'progressive overload' and it's a very important principle for getting results.

A note for beginners – I suggest that you stay on the beginner workout plan for 12 weeks, increasing only the weight or the repetitions as you feel your body is ready (remember that you will know if you're ready to progress when your body can execute more than the suggested repetitions, with perfect form). After the 12 weeks you will most likely feel you can take on more difficult variations – this is when I would suggest attempting the advanced programme. Again, correct form is always key, check your moves in the mirror or record yourself if you're not sure of what to do. The beauty of social media is that you can always share your videos and ask me for some tips.

A note for advanced movers – You will most likely be able to determine when your body needs more challenge, however the same general rules apply. Increase the weight or the repetitions, however do not try to change both variables at the same time – it's one or the other. Strong and elegant execution is always the best indication of whether or not we should be progressing. If you're unable to perform the movement as it is, then there is no need to increase the intensity or volume.

At the end of the 28 days – I encourage you to pick the book up and use it as a reference. If your motivation to lift dwindles, I guarantee that reading about 'the booty' will get your butt back into gear (pun intended). If your meditation practice becomes a little sporadic, open up to page 87 where I discuss the scientifically proven benefits of meditation. If you suddenly feel like you couldn't possibly eat another green vegetable, then go and buy a doughnut but have a read of why your body needs macro- and micronutrients. Education is the BEST motivation. When we understand how and why something benefits us, we will do it more. This book is going to be your secret weapon to maintain that motivation for 28 days and beyond. And the more you continue to develop a balance of strength and flexibility and nourishment of the body and mind, the more you will fall in love with a 'healthy lifestyle'. It's that love and enjoyment that will have you lifting, lengthening and nourishing for the rest of your life.

FORMULAS FOR GEEKS (LIKE ME)

This section contains some of the formulas that are required to understand your approximate basal metabolic rate (BMR) as well as your approximate total daily energy expenditure (TDEE). I say approximate, because without some hefty and sophisticated equipment measuring your heart rate and body composition, it can be pretty tricky to get an accurate amount. However, this does give you a ballpark figure and allows you to be aware of what might be more ideal for your body. It by no means is the encouragement for you to start aggressively counting calories or scanning every ingredient into MyFitnessPal app in an effort to stay under or above these numbers. It is simply so that you can be more self-aware of your body's requirements.

First we need to calculate your BMR. This gives us the amount of calories your body requires to function without any exercise or movement. Basically, if you were to just lie there all day, in order to maintain your current body weight you would need to consume this many calories.

To calculate BMR I use the **Mifflin St. Jeor Equation:**

For men: BMR = 10 x weight (kg) + 6.25 x height (cm) – 5 x age (years) + 5
For women: BMR = 10 x weight (kg) + 6.25 x height (cm) – 5 x age (years) – 161

Next you will need to calculate your TDEE, which basically looks at your daily activity levels.

TDEE = BMR x PAL (physical activity level)

Physical activity levels are based on studies [20] and literature reviewed by the scientific advisory committee on nutrition, but given the many variables associated with each person's lifestyle, it is very difficult to find an accurate number that will fit all of our bodies and lifestyle situations. The point of this formula was to give you a ballpark figure so that you were a little more aware of what may be required for your body.

On my plan you will be training just under 6 hours per week, so the formula accommodating for this kind of activity level is approximately as follows:

BMR x 1.375 = TDEE

For example, if my BMR was 1100kcal, the formula and result would look like this:

1100kcal x 1.375 = 1512.5kcal

So in order for me to maintain my current weight, I would need to consume 1512kcal per day. Remember – these are very basic and potentially flawed calculations. As I have already mentioned, calories are not the be all and end all of developing a healthy body; nutrient quality and quantity is paramount. However, it can be interesting to have a little more understanding on what your body requires.

GLOSSARY

alcohol metabolisation The digestive processing of alcohol within the body and predominantly the liver. Ethanol is a poison to the body and is therefore promptly metabolised via the use of two enzymes: alcohol dehydrogenase and aldehyde dehydrogenase. These help the body to break down the alcohol molecule, which enables us to eliminate it from the body. (National Institute of Alcoholic Abuse, 2007)

alignment In the case of weight training, this refers to the placement of your body in relation to a force (gravity and your body or gravity and a weight). Poor alignment and posture while training can result in muscular imbalances, eventually leading to dysfunctional movement and potentially pain. Good alignment of the body enables healthy biomechanics (see below) and will allow you to strengthen the body without further impairment or damage to the joints or muscles.

amino acids The human body has thousands of different proteins, all of which are necessary for functioning properly and staying alive; amino acids are the building blocks of these proteins. While the body can produce certain amino acids, there are nine essential ones that it cannot produce itself and therefore we need to obtain them from external food sources. Those essential amino acids are: histidine, isoleucine, leucine, lysine, methionine, phenylalanine, threonine, tryptophan and valine. Eating a range of different coloured and types of foods ensures that you obtain these different amino acids, essential for life and efficient functioning of your body.

bioavailability The degree to which any given substance to enter the bloodstream is able to be used by the body. For example, whey is easily absorbed and used by the body so has a high bioavailability and is therefore an optimal protein source.

biomechanics The study of the mechanical laws relating to the movement or structure of living organisms.

Bosu A piece of fitness equipment that is essentially like a Swiss ball or exercise ball that has been cut in half and given a stable, firm base. The title is based on an acronym: 'both sides utilised'. It is most effective for core training, however, I do not recommend that you perform deadlifts or squats on an unstable surface, with research showing that it yields no further muscular activation than performing it on a stable ground and could actually be more dangerous.

central nervous system The collection of tissues responsible for controlling activities within the body. It processes information received from all parts, as well as the environment around the body.

cortisol A hormone within the body that reacts to and is released in times of stress. What is important to remember is that many things can cause stress, from arguments with our lovers to deadlines from our bosses, in fact, even exercise is a form of stress on the body. Excessive levels of stress, therefore excessive levels of the hormone cortisol, can be extremely detrimental to the body, in many cases being the reason for stubborn belly fat. While practising meditation and yoga won't pay the bills or fix your problems immediately, they will enable you to lower those cortisol levels, which in turn will support your body (and your health and fitness goals).

deep core This term is usually referring to your transverse abdominus (or TVA) which is the corset-like structure originating at the thoracolumbar spine (middle back), wrapping around the organs, and attaching to the linea alba (the fiborous line of ligaments that runs along your abdomen, separating your six-pack) and pubic crest (at the front of your pelvis). This muscle does not flex the trunk, instead it serves as support for the abdominal organs, and also helps to compress the rib cage in breathing. It also aids in stability of the spine and pelvis. Many people can have a strong rectus abdominus (six-pack) while having a weak transverse abdominus, however this is not ideal and can lead to malalignment and poor stability of the spine.

'gainz' Refers to achieving muscular development from lifting weight and eating foods, e.g. 'woah – have you been doing something different in your workouts? Look at those amazing arms gainz.'

HIIT The acronym for High Intensity Interval Training. It refers to a type of training in which you perform short, intense bursts of exercise, followed by short intervals of rest.

Hypertrophy Defined as increased volume of tissue in the body. When I mention hypertrophy I'm referring to the growth and increased volume of muscle tissue, however you can use it in the context of organs too.

MCT oil Saturated fats are quite diverse in their structure; they comprise short-chain, medium-chain and long-chain triglycerides (fatty acids), and each influences the body in a different way. MCTs – medium chain triglycerides, can be broken down and digested by the body much faster than LCTs (long-chain triglycerides).

MCT oil is a combination of coconut oil and palm oil (which should be sustainably sourced). It can be digested and utilised by the body more like a carbohydrate than fat, which means it is ideal for providing quick burning energy. There are also some studies to suggest that it might aid in weight loss or weight management.

Myofascial Refers to skeletal muscle and its surrounding fascia.

Proprioception The sensory feedback and information that is used by the body in order to gain an understanding of joint movement and positioning. For example, a gymnast must have exceptional proprioception in order to execute fast and intense movements, while also maintaining good stability when required. Good proprioception helps us to move more efficiently and safely.

Trapezius A large superficial muscle that is located in the posterior thorax and neck.

TRX Referred to as suspension training, the TRX is a long strap with two arms that is usually hung from a ceiling or door frame. The arms have two handles that you hold onto or even slip your feet into, enabling you to work with your body weight in various ways. A common exercise would be a bodyweight row in which you stand firmly, hold onto the handles and lean back. From there you would pull your chest to the handles using the muscles of your arms and upper back, thereby resisting your body weight.

WORKS CITED

Beauchamp, Gary K., et al. 'Phytochemistry: ibuprofen-like activity in extra-virgin olive oil.' *Nature* 437.7055 (2005): 45–46.

Borota, Daniel, et al. 'Post-study caffeine administration enhances memory consolidation in humans.' *Nature Neuroscience* 17.2 (2014): 201–203.

Bowen, J., M. Noakes, and P. M. Clifton. 'Appetite hormones and energy intake in obese men after consumption of fructose, glucose and whey protein beverages.' *International Journal of Obesity* 31.11 (2007): 1696–1703.

Bradley, Una, et al. 'Low-fat versus low-carbohydrate weight reduction diets.' *Diabetes* 58.12 (2009): 2741–2748.

Davidson, Richard J., et al. 'Alterations in brain and immune function produced by mindfulness meditation.' *Psychosomatic Medicine* 65.4 (2003): 564–570.

El Asmar, Margueritta S., Joseph J. Naoum, and Elias J. Arbid. 'Vitamin k dependent proteins and the role of vitamin k2 in the modulation of vascular calcification: a review.' *Oman Medical Journal* 29.3 (2014): 172–177.

Eskelinen, Marjo H., and Miia Kivipelto. 'Caffeine as a protective factor in dementia and Alzheimer's disease.' *Journal of Alzheimer's Disease* 20.S1 (2010): 167–174.

Groen, Bart, et al. 'Protein ingestion before sleep improves postexercise overnight recovery.' *Medicine and Science in Sports and Exercise* 44.8 (2012): 1560–1569.

Hagerman, Fredrick C., et al. 'Effects of high-intensity resistance training on untrained older men. I. Strength, cardiovascular, and metabolic responses.' *The Journals of Gerontology Series A: Biological Sciences and Medical Sciences* 55.7 (2000): B336–B346.

Hoffman, Jay R., et al. 'Effect of nutritionally enriched coffee consumption on aerobic and anaerobic exercise performance.' *The Journal of Strength and Conditioning Research* 21.2 (2007): 456–459.

Holten, Mads K., et al. 'Strength training increases insulin-mediated glucose uptake, GLUT4 content, and insulin signaling in skeletal muscle in patients with type 2 diabetes.' *Diabetes* 53.2 (2004): 294–305.

Layne, Jennifer E., and Miriam E. Nelson. 'The effects of progressive resistance training on bone density: a review.' *Medicine and Science in Sports and Exercise* 31.1 (1999): 25–30.

Luders, Eileen, et al. 'The underlying anatomical correlates of long-term meditation: larger hippocampal and frontal volumes of gray matter.' *Neuroimage* 45.3 (2009): 672–678.

Maia, L., and A. De Mendonça. 'Does caffeine intake protect from Alzheimer's disease?' *European Journal of Neurology* 9.4 (2002): 377–382.

Ramel, Wiveka, et al. 'The effects of mindfulness meditation on cognitive processes and affect in patients with past depression.' *Cognitive Therapy and Research* 28.4 (2004): 433–455.

Schoenfeld, Brad J. 'The mechanisms of muscle hypertrophy and their application to resistance training.' *The Journal of Strength and Conditioning Research* 24.10 (2010): 2857–2872.

Scientific Advisory Committee on Nutrition. *Dietary Reference Values for Energy* (2011). Retrieved from: https://www.gov.uk/government/uploads/system/uploads/attachment_data/file/339317/SACN_Dietary_Reference_Values_for_Energy.pdf

Singh, Nalin A., Karen M. Clements, and Maria A. Fiatarone. 'A randomized controlled trial of progressive resistance training in depressed elders.' *The Journals of Gerontology Series A: Biological Sciences and Medical Sciences* 52.1 (1997): M27–M35.

The British Dietetic Association. *Food Fact Sheet: Wholegrains* (2016).

Willoughby, D. S., J. R. Stout, and C. D. Wilborn. 'Effects of resistance training and protein plus amino acid supplementation on muscle anabolism, mass, and strength.' *Amino Acids* 32.4 (2007): 467–477.

REFERENCES

1. Hagerman, F.C., 1999

2. Layne, J.E., 1999

3. Holten, M.K., 2004

4. Singh, N.A., 1996

5. Schoenfeld, D.B., 2010

6. Schoenfeld, D.B., 2010

7. Commonwealth Scientific and Industrial Research Organisation, Human Nutrition, Adelaide, Australia, 2007

8. (Exercise and Biochemical Nutrition Laboratory, Baylor University, Waco, Texas, 2007; Commonwealth Scientific and Industrial Research Organisation, Human Nutrition, Adelaide, Australia, 2007

9. Department of Human Movement Sciences, NUTRIM School for Nutrition, Toxicology and Metabolism, Maastricht University Medical Centre+, Maastricht, The Netherlands, 2012

10. British Dietetic Association, 2016

11. Regional Centre for Endocrinology and Diabetes, Royal Victoria Hospital, Belfast, U.K.; 2Nutrition and Metabolism Group, The Queen's University of Belfast, Belfast, U.K. Corresponding author: Steven J. Hunter, 2009

12. Beauchamp, G.K. et al., 2005

13. Borota, D., 2014

14. Maia, L., 2002

15. Eskelinen, M.H., 20105

16. Hoffman, J. R. et al., 2007

17. Ramel, W., 2004

18. Luders, E., 2009

19. Davidson, R.J., 2003

20. Scientific Advisory Committee on Nutrition, 2011

INDEX

INDEX

INDEX

INDEX

INDEX